PCOS

A Step-By-Step Guide to Reverse Polycystic Ovary Syndrome, Balance Your Hormones, Boost Your Metabolism, & Restore Your Fertility

Jessica Olson

© **Copyright 2019 - All rights reserved.**

The content contained within this book may not be reproduced, duplicated or transmitted without direct written permission from the author or the publisher.

Under no circumstances will any blame or legal responsibility be held against the publisher, or author, for any damages, reparation, or monetary loss due to the information contained within this book. Either directly or indirectly.

Legal Notice:

This book is copyright protected. This book is only for personal use. You cannot amend, distribute, sell, use, quote or paraphrase any part, or the content within this book, without the consent of the author or publisher.

Disclaimer Notice:

Please note the information contained within this document is for educational and entertainment purposes only. All effort has been executed to present accurate, up to date, and reliable, complete information. No warranties of any kind are declared or implied. Readers acknowledge that the author is not engaging in the rendering of legal, financial, medical or professional advice. The content within this book has been derived from various sources. Please consult a licensed professional before attempting any techniques outlined in this book.

By reading this document, the reader agrees that under no circumstances is the author responsible for any losses, direct or indirect, which are incurred as a result of the use of information contained within this document, including, but not limited to, — errors, omissions, or inaccuracies.

Table of Contents

Introduction: Getting to Know More About PCOS 1

Chapter 1: What Causes PCOS and What Are the Symptoms 5

   Symptoms of PCOS in Women 8

   Does PCOS Mean Miscarriages? 14

   What to Do Once Diagnosed with PCOS 16

   Can PCOS Be Prevented? 19

Chapter 2: Diet and Lifestyle with PCOS 21

   Best Types of Exercise for PCOS 26

   Nutrition for PCOS 27

Chapter 3: Treatments for PCOS 34

   Other Herbs for PCOS Treatments 38

   Medical Treatments for PCOS 41

   Reducing Other PCOS Symptoms with Medications 45

Chapter 4: Getting Pregnant with PCOS 48

   Diets for Boosting Fertility 53

   Fertility Foods 59

   Gluten-Free for Fertility 64

Vitamin Supplements for Pregnancy 66

Bad Habits and Fertility 70

Chapter 5: Menopause and PCOS *74*

Chapter 6: Birth Control and PCOS *85*

Long-term Side Effects of Birth Control 90

Alternatives to Birth Control Pills 92

Best Birth Control Pills for PCOS 96

Chapter 7: Research on PCOS *100*

Relationship Between AMH and PCOS 102

PCOS and IVF 106

Other Fertility Treatments for Women with PCOS 110

Fertilization Surgeries for Women with PCOS 114

Conclusion *123*

Self-Esteem Problems with PCOS 129

PCOS And Relationships 132

Introduction: Getting to Know More About PCOS

PCOS means polycystic ovary syndrome. It is a type of disorder of the hormones and is very common in women who are in the ages of reproduction. This could start as early as twenty years old and go up to 45 years old. Women have even been diagnosed with it while they were still in puberty. This disorder does affect quite a few women. In fact, one in ten women are affected by it.

PCOS is very common, as you can see. It is treatable and can be a cause of infertility and painful periods. The hormonal imbalance of PCOS can create major problems in the ovaries. The ovaries help to produce the eggs that women need in order to conceive a baby. When women have PCOS, the egg could not develop as it should during ovulation and this can begin to cause problems for women.

There are four different types of PCOS. They all have different effects on women, but most of them do have the same treatments and symptoms. The first type of PCOS is called Insulin-resistant PCOS. This is a type of PCOS that is generally caused by sugar, trans fat, smoking cigarettes, and pollution. This type of PCOS triggers the ovaries to produce more testosterone instead of estrogen. The best way to get rid of this type of PCOS is to stop eating and drinking sugar altogether. There are small amounts of sugar that can be healthy for the body, but too much will cause this type of PCOS. Doctors can also recommend taking inositol for about six to nine months.

Another type of PCOS is called Pill-induced PCOS. This is one of the most common types of PCOS and it will generally develop when women take birth control. The birth control pills can inhibit ovulation in women. These effects can last much longer after women stop using birth control in order to become pregnant. Many women will not begin to ovulate normally for many years after they have stopped using the pill. When women have periods that are happening before their normal cycle, they may have Pill-induced PCOS. When doctors run blood tests on these women, they tend to have a higher level of LH.

Inflammatory PCOS is caused by inflammation of the body. This inflammation could begin in the ovaries but can also occur in other places internally. When a woman has unbalanced hormones, androgens get produced and PCOS can begin. This inflammation can be caused by quite a few factors. Stress, inflammatory diets, and toxins can cause the inflammation that causes this type of PCOS. Generally, women who have a gluten intolerance can be diagnosed with this type of

PCOS. There are multiple symptoms of this type of PCOS such as headaches, skin allergies, and infections. When blood tests are taken, a vitamin D deficiency can be picked up. Doctors will suggest taking supplements of magnesium and vitamin D when this is diagnosed.

Hidden PCOS is the fourth type of PCOS. This type of PCOS is fairly easy to get rid of. It takes about three to five months for it to be treated and it is usually caused by thyroid disease, lack of iodine (the ovaries do need iodine), a vegetarian diet, and using artificial sweeteners and sugars. Vegetarian diets can cause this type of PCOS because of the lack of zinc in this type of diet and the ovaries function best when they have heavier amounts of zinc. This type of PCOS is one that many doctors will suggest natural treatments for. A diet change is one of the easiest ways to resolve this type of PCOS.

In this book, we will explain the causes and symptoms of PCOS, how to treat it, how it can cause infertility, and how you can still get pregnant even though you have PCOS. This is not a disorder that should keep you from trying to get pregnant, but it should help to inspire you to seek the treatments and talk to your doctor about safe ways to get pregnant with PCOS. This book will also share a lot of important information about what women can expect when they are diagnosed with PCOS. There are a lot of things that doctors will not tell women when they have been diagnosed. For example, not many doctors will dwell on the fact that women with PCOS may develop depression and may start to feel less than adequate. This is a completely natural way to feel and we will explain how to combat these feelings as well.

Chapter 1: What Causes PCOS and What Are the Symptoms

PCOS has recently been shown to occur in many more women than ever before. Doctors are concerned about this heavy rate of women being exposed to it and how it changes their entire body. The causes of it are clear, although, some women never know they have it until it is too late. There are a few causes that have been found, but in some cases, doctors are not sure what causes PCOS.

Having heightened levels of androgens can cause it. These hormones are sometimes referred to as male hormones. Women do have smaller amounts of androgens in their bodies already, but when the amount of these hormones increases, PCOS can occur. These androgens control many things in the bodies of men, such as baldness. When women have too many androgens, they may start to hold in the eggs that should be released during the menstrual cycle. These androgens can also cause acne and extra hair growth. These are two of the signs that a woman may have PCOS.

A higher number of androgens can also intervene with the communication from the brain during ovulation. This can cause the body to produce eggs, but not to release them as ovulation generally occurs. If a woman is trying to get pregnant during this time, it can change up the whole process. This can also cause cysts to form in the ovaries that can mature and grow. This can cause types of ovarian cancer and infertility.

Another cause of PCOS is having higher levels of insulin. Insulin is a hormone in the body that controls how our food is turned into energy. Some people have insulin resistance and that is when the cells in our bodies do not respond commonly to insulin. This is what causes the amount of insulin in our bodies to be higher than it should be. Women with PCOS with higher levels of insulin, may notice that they have gained weight and become obese, that their eating habits have changed and become unhealthy, they are not getting enough exercise, or they have a history in their family of diabetes. If the body continues to be resistant to insulin, type 2 diabetes may develop over time.

Genetics also seems to be a common cause of PCOS. A woman's genes seem to be quite the trigger for PCOS. Even though this is a new disease, doctors and scientists have found that women, who had mothers with PCOS, are 25% more likely to be diagnosed with it. They are about 33% more likely to have it if their sister has PCOS. Because our genes determine so much of our health, women with these abnormalities should be aware that it is important to give other women in the family the knowledge if anything has been seen as abnormal.

There have been some genetic studies recently that have shown that there is a gene that can play a huge role in the development of PCOS. This news is coming from PCOS doctors and it is exciting to see the progress in the studies of it. This could be a huge breakthrough when it comes to finding a cure for the disorder. Through different genetic tests, doctors have now found that one or two genes in women could cause the disorder. This study took place this year and tests 60 families. In these families, at least one of them had PCOS. There were genetic tests done on the families and these tests were done to see what genes one family had and the others did not. It was found that some of the genes had variations that could possibly be the cause of PCOS and others did not. One of the results was a rare genetic variant called DENND1A. The variations in this study varied from family to family, but the doctors think that this is one of the genes that could be the main cause of PCOS. It is now the goal of these doctors to find out just how to stop this gene from being spread from parent to child. There may be ways to manipulate the gene, but it is not certain yet if it can be done.

Although we still don't have a cure for PCOS, this study is a huge breakthrough in the research being done to help fight it. The doctors feel that it is a great step in the right direction. The doctors are excited to see a small correlation in the spreading of PCOS in the family. They now may have a specific gene that spreads it and now it is up to them to do more research on how to fight this one gene. This could be a new screening that doctors can do if the research shows more positive signs of this gene. We know that we are excited to share this information with women who have PCOS. Perhaps in the next few years, doctors will be able to find the gene and mutate or change it in order to keep women from having PCOS.

With most of the causes of PCOS being known, it is also important that women know what the symptoms are. Women need to be aware of what they are going through in order to keep up with their health. If a woman is trying to have a baby, the symptoms can change up the process and they may need more help from their doctors. Here are some of the symptoms of PCOS and how to combat them.

Symptoms of PCOS in Women

Because of how new this disease is, a lot of women don't know that they even have PCOS. The symptoms will generally show up around the time of puberty and can even start to develop later on in life. Some of the symptoms do go unnoticed, so it is important for women to get their screenings each year and be open with their doctors about the changes occurring in their bodies.

One of the main symptoms of PCOS is having missed or irregular periods. When a woman misses a period, their first thought maybe that they are pregnant. This is also a big sign of PCOS, especially if they are missing their periods multiple times a year. This is when a period tracker is good for a woman to have. A period tracker is a calendar that helps women to follow their periods month by month. Many women who are trying to have a child use it to track their ovulation days, but it is a good tool for any woman to have.

When a woman misses a period or it is irregular, this can cause cysts to develop on the ovaries. Cysts on the ovaries can cause infertility and cancer. Painful periods are another cause of cysts in the ovaries. Along with painful periods, women may notice too much hair on their face, upper back, and chest area. They may also start to notice that their hair is starting to get thinner in some spots. Lastly, the appearance of skin tags around the neck or armpits may begin. All of these are sure signs of PCOS.

There are some other signs that women may notice, but don't think too much of it. These signs are mood swings, which some people will blame on PMS or mental health issues. A lot of women don't realize that there could possibly more going on than they think. PCOS can cause these mood swings, along with depression and anxiety. If these mood swings become worse, it is a great idea for a woman to see her doctor to be sure that PCOS is not what is causing them.

Another symptom that PCOS brings is pelvic pain. This pain doesn't seem to be consistent, but it seems to come around during the time when periods should occur and it can also bring very heavy bleeding with it. Women can have problems with this pain when they are not menstruating as well.

Headaches and sleep issues are two other symptoms of PCOS. Headaches are generally caused during changes in hormones and if a woman is already having problems with her hormones, this can make the headaches greater and even turn them into migraines. Insomnia and other sleep problems can be caused by PCOS too. Many doctors have linked PCOS with sleep apnea.

These symptoms may seem small in the grand scheme of things, but if they are happening regularly, a woman needs to take them seriously and go check in with her doctor. Even if it ends up not being PCOS, she will at least have some peace of mind about what is happening with her body.

Unfortunately, there are some symptoms of PCOS that women may not have seen or even known that they had. These are called the silent signs. PCOS is under-diagnosed more than we think it is. There is about ten percent of women who are affected by PCOS and have no idea that they are. Their doctors have misdiagnosed the disorder and have told women that they have something else. It is the most common of the hormone disorders in women of reproductive age and this could be part of the reason that doctors don't know how to diagnose it. There are women who have had it their entire lives and no one has ever diagnosed it as PCOS. Because the symptoms do vary for each woman, it is important that doctors know the silent signs as well.

Missing periods is one of the most common silent signs. Generally if a woman is trying to have a child, missing a period is a blessing for her. That is, until she realizes that she is not pregnant, she just has PCOS. For women, ovulation is key in order to have a child. If a woman misses her periods, she will find herself unsure of her ovulation cycle. Irregular periods are also a silent sign that she may have PCOS. Stress levels and weight gain can be two of the reasons for missing periods.

As women age, they will start to notice a random hair popping up on their face. Many women think this is natural and normal as they enter their mid- '30s to late '40s. It doesn't have to be normal because it could be a silent sign of PCOS. This a common sign of PCOS and when women begin to develop more hair on their face, it is called hirsutism. This causes larger amounts of dark and coarse hair on the face of women. It can also grow on their chests and backs. Generally it is thought of as a genetic issue, but it can happen because of the larger amounts of androgens in the body. This occurs in PCOS patients. There are some complications that arise from hirsutism. Women can become emotionally damaged because they have become very self-conscious about the extra hair on their bodies. There are no physical complications, but for women who have PCOS, this extra hair growth becomes a worry for them.

Another silent sign for PCOS is acne and other skin problems. Many women have never had acne problems until they were diagnosed with PCOS. Some of these women think that they are just having acne break out because their periods are starting, but with PCOS, acne can start up again at any time. Generally the acne will begin to form along the jawline. This type of acne is pretty resistant to medications and will pass with time. The breakouts may become more rampant and eventually they more turn into skin tags. Skin tags can be taken care of with medications and some people will use tea tree oil to combat skin tags. Tea tree oil will cause skin tags to dry up and then they will fall off. The sooner that these medications can be applied to the skin tags, the quicker they will fall off of the skin. Skin tags aren't dangerous, but many women with PCOS get very embarrassed by the number of skin tags that have formed on their face and neck. They can also form in the armpits and chest.

Sleep apnea is another silent sign of PCOS. It is linked to PCOS because it leads to high blood pressure, mood swings, and obesity. All of these are signs of PCOS as well. PCOS patients are more likely to develop breathing problems when they are sleeping because of their weight gain. Their insulin resistance is another reason that sleep apnea can occur as well. How do women know if they have sleep apnea? They will usually snore very loudly and feel exhausted even though they got eight hours of sleep or more. Doctors have some great ways to help with sleep disorders such as sleep apnea.

Some of the ways to get better sleep include meditation exercises, developing a new sleep routine, changing pillows, eating a banana before bed, taking a bath before bedtime, sleeping in comfortable clothing, making sure the bedroom is painted in a cooling and soothing color, and turning off devices at bedtime. Lights can cause problems with sleep routines so it is important to have the room as dark as possible. Also, women with PCOS will need to know that they should not eat a big meal before bed.

If doctors have found ovarian cysts in women, they may have PCOS. Ovarian cysts can form in any woman. They are not always dangerous, but most of them do need to be removed from a woman's ovaries. Many women that have been diagnosed with PCOS have ovarian cysts. These cysts are part of the reason that many women cannot get pregnant because the cysts stall ovulation and that can halt pregnancy. Young women are more prone to have these cysts. Older women will seldom have them in their ovaries.

It is important for women to know all of the signs of PCOS. Once they have been diagnosed, then they will need to talk to their doctor about just what is next for them.

Does PCOS Mean Miscarriages?

Quite a few women are concerned that when they are diagnosed with PCOS, they may end up having more miscarriages. It is not uncommon at all for women to worry about this, in fact, it is one of the main worries that women with PCOS have. PCOS does make it very difficult for women to get pregnant and there are studies that show that it can increase miscarriages in women. With PCOS and fertility treatments, the odds of having a miscarriage actually go up.

Doctors have said that the risk of miscarriages can go down if the diet and lifestyle changes. There are medications for PCOS that can also make these chances go down. It is very important that if a woman with PCOS has had a miscarriage already, she needs to make her doctor aware of that. She may have increased chances of having more miscarriages after that.

It is not a possibility to prevent miscarriages, but there are ways that women can try. Diet and exercise are one way and taking care of the body is another. Doctors can give their patients with PCOS the best guidance in order to help them take care of their body and their baby. Most of the time miscarriages occur because of genetic abnormalities.

Women who are at risk of having a high-risk pregnancy also need to talk to their doctors about possible miscarriages. Most doctors will put their high-risk patients on bed rest after a certain number of weeks. Doctors want their patients to have a healthy pregnancy so they have quite a few suggestions to help them get through the entire pregnancy. There are so many ways for women to have a healthy pregnancy and their doctors can help them every step of the way!

What to Do Once Diagnosed with PCOS

As more research is being done on PCOS and how to diagnose, many women are growing concerned that this could be something they are suffering with. Currently, the tests for PCOS come from full medical exams, blood tests, pelvic exams, and pap smears. There is not one test that can determine PCOS in a woman, but researchers are working diligently on finding one. These tests can be frustrating for women because it is hard to determine if their symptoms are PCOS or something else.

Doctors are moving forward with trying to confirm a woman's symptoms as PCOS. There have been quite a few problems when it comes time to diagnose PCOS. Women must go through a series of tests in order to see if they do have PCOS. There are blood tests, pap smears, and physicals that they must take. Even then, many doctors are not quite sure that they have PCOS. This is why researchers are working extremely hard on making one test that will diagnose PCOS.

The physical exam will show the doctor the levels of androgens in a woman's body, excessive hair growth, or acne on their body. There will be a pelvic exam at this time to see if there are any cysts on the ovaries, and the doctor will check the weight of the patient. All of these factors will help them to determine if the woman does have PCOS.

The blood tests will include some imaging tests as well. These blood tests will show the doctor the levels of hormones in the woman's body. There will be a pelvic ultrasound during this time as well and this will help to get a closer look at the ovaries.

Once patients have been diagnosed with PCOS, they may be unsure what to do next. Their doctor will give them a lot of information on how to take care of themselves during this time. The treatment that the doctor chooses for the patient depends on the condition of the PCOS. One of the first treatments that the doctor may suggest is a complete lifestyle and diet change.

We have touched on the things that women should do when they have been diagnosed with PCOS, but what about the things they shouldn't do? There are many things that women shouldn't do when they are made aware of their PCOS diagnosis. One of these is smoke cigarettes. Smoking can increase the chances of heart disease, diabetes, and other health problems.

Eating high sugar foods is another thing that women shouldn't do when they are diagnosed with PCOS. These foods can cause problems with insulin resistance and can make symptoms of PCOS even worse. Avoiding sugars is key when a woman is diagnosed with PCOS. By focusing on more natural sugars, women can help their bodies once they have been diagnosed with PCOS.

Exercise is key after being diagnosed with PCOS. It may be fun to lay on the couch and watch television all day, but this will do nothing for weight loss and a healthier lifestyle. It isn't hard to get outside and take a walk or go to the park and go for a jog. Lifting weights at home or exercising with a kettlebell are great ideas for those colder or rainy days at home.

Women shouldn't forget to log their periods when they have been diagnosed with PCOS. By keeping up with the cycles, they will be able to confirm if their periods are regular or irregular. This information is important to their doctor to help them determine if they are able to get pregnant. There are special apps that women can download that will help them keep track, even when they are too busy to write it down.

Some women get diagnosed with PCOS and immediately go into a denial stage. There is no reason to ignore the symptoms of PCOS. Ignoring them doesn't make them go away and cannot help the condition any. There are medical treatment options and once a woman has been diagnosed, it is important that she knows what to do. If she feels scared, it is a good idea for her to check in with her doctor and express her feelings with them.

Can PCOS Be Prevented?

Women all over the world want to know if they can actually prevent PCOS from happening to them. As of right now, the answer is no, but there is a lot of evidence that there may be a cure soon. There have to be two conditions present in a woman in order to diagnose her with PCOS. Here are a few of the conditions:

- Irregular periods that are chronic
- High levels of male hormones
- Small cysts on the ovaries
- Absent periods

PCOS cannot entirely be prevented, but there is more and more evidence pointing that we can halt it. The research being done in the world of genetics has shown us that some genes do need to be present in order for PCOS to develop. Once those genes are present, the woman may be diagnosed with PCOS, but what if scientists could isolate that gene and disrupt it? Would this be a way to prevent PCOS from occurring altogether? We think so. We just need to keep an eye on all of the research that is being done now on PCOS. Scientists are well on their way to finding out what can help prevent it.

Genetics does have a lot to do with diabetes and other health-related issues that occur with PCOS. It can be passed down on the mother and father's side and there are signs that women may develop it in the future. Diabetes, obesity, and poor diet are all factors that are handed down to women in their genes or in their family life. Many of these factors can be changed by the woman, but she has to work really hard in order to do so.

The impact of PCOS can be lessened though. A healthy lifestyle is one way to do it, but women can also exercise and begin a birth control regiment. Taking medications for diabetes can also help to lessen the effects of PCOS.

Chapter 2: Diet and Lifestyle with PCOS

When a woman is diagnosed with PCOS, they must make some lifestyle and diet changes in order to make sure their body starts to heal. One of the major symptoms of PCOS is having insulin resistance. This means that the body doesn't process the hormone insulin in the body in the correct way. Insulin helps to provide the body with energy that it gets from foods. It also helps to control the blood sugar in the body. Women with PCOS may need to lower their sugar levels in order to keep their insulin balanced.

When the suggestion is made that they do eat less sugar, the doctor will also suggest lowering the carbohydrate intact. There are some healthier carbohydrates that contain natural sugars such as fish, vegetables, and fruits. Doctors will also suggest eating more grains that are high in fiber. This is just the first step for women who have been diagnosed with PCOS. The foods that are high in fiber help with controlling the blood sugar levels in the body.

In order to maintain a healthy diet that helps the blood sugar, women with PCOS should avoid eating refined carbohydrates, white flour, rice, potatoes, sugary drinks, soda, juice, and other sugary treats.

Women with PCOS should add some green vegetables to their diets such as broccoli, spinach, and kale. These vegetables are high in fiber and help with the insulin in the body and the blood sugar levels. Lean proteins, such as fish can also help greatly. It is important that women with PCOS also eat foods that are anti-inflammatory. A couple of these are turmeric and tomatoes.

High fiber foods are very important in the diet of women with PCOS. Along with broccoli, cauliflower, and Brussels sprouts make great options to add to the diet. Green and red peppers, beans, lentils, almonds, berries, sweet potatoes, winter squash, and pumpkin are also great vegetables that are high in fiber and can help women that are diagnosed with PCOS. The foods that are considered anti-inflammatory are kale, spinach, walnuts, olive oil, strawberries, blueberries, fatty fish like salmon and sardines, and tofu.

There are many foods to avoid when being diagnosed with PCOS as well. Foods high in carbohydrates need to be taken out of the diet, sugary snacks and drinks, red meats, white bread, muffins, pastries for breakfast, desserts, white potatoes, and foods that are made with white flour. Reading the labels on foods can really help to change up the diet. There are ingredients that women need to look out for when shopping and they are sucrose, high fructose corn syrup, and dextrose.

Along with the changing of the diet, women with PCOS need to be aware that they may need to change their lifestyle altogether. One of the first lifestyle changes that doctors will recommend is losing or managing weight. Many of the women with PCOS are considered overweight for their age and height. This could turn into obesity and it could also lead to health problems. The health problems caused by obesity include type 2 diabetes, infertility, and heart disease. There are nutritionists that are available to create a healthier diet for women with PCOS. It is important to count calories and portion sizes when weight gain has occurred. Portion size is key when it comes to losing weight!

Exercise is another lifestyle change that doctors will recommend. There are quite a few exercises that doctors do recommend for battling PCOS and losing weight. Physical activity as a whole is great for women's fertility and it helps to lower disease risks. Many women who are obese feel that starting exercises could hurt their body more than it helps them. This is far from the truth. These women can start slow with going on walks and even jumping jacks or jumping rope. Stationary bike riding is also a great way to lose weight when starting out.

For fighting obesity and PCOS, it is suggested that women get about 150 minutes a week of exercise. Basically, aiming for a solid 30 minutes a day of exercise is what it takes to get some of the weight off. Once the body is moving differently and on a regular basis, the weight will begin to come off and come off quicker each time the exercises are done. This will not happen overnight, so it is important that women continue these exercises until they are at the weight best for their height and age.

Cardio exercises are a great way of reducing insulin resistance and boosting fertility. They can also work as a mood stabilizer. Cardio exercises vary from brisk walking to swimming and cycling. Jogging and brisk walking are also cardio exercises. These exercises reduce chances of heart disease and type 2 diabetes. It is important to do at least 30 minutes of these exercises each day to begin to see results. Cardio activities can boost the mood greatly and can also help improve the menstrual cycle and ovulation in women.

Strength training is another type of exercise that works well for women with PCOS. This is also a good way to reduce insulin resistance and increase metabolism. This helps to perk up the body's composition and manage weight. These exercises vary from push-ups, squats, and dips and help to boost the ways that insulin functions in the body. This can also boost metabolism and build muscle mass in the body.

High-intensity interval training is another way to help women with PCOS. This is a great way to increase cardiovascular fitness in general and helps to build a smaller waist and healthier BMI. When women burn a lot of calories through high-intensity interval training, they will begin to notice changes very quickly. These exercises have helped women achieve their goal weight and have seen about a 10 to 15% weight loss since they began. These exercises help to reduce the testosterone in a woman's body, which makes her more likely to fight off the symptoms of PCOS.

Core strengthening is another way to prepare the body for being pregnant. Most women are not prepared to the fullest for pregnancy, but these exercises are part of to do so. These core exercises can help to strengthen the muscles in the spine and keep from getting injured during exercise. Core exercises can also be used to help to train the pelvic floor muscles. This is very important when wanting to have a child. When these exercises are used, sexual health can be boosted, pelvic stability improves, and women can start to prevent incontinence. All of these will add up to make a healthy and happy pregnancy.

Best Types of Exercise for PCOS

We have described the various forms of exercises that can help with PCOS, but there are many other ways to do so. One of these is by walking. This is one of the best ways to help with PCOS because all a woman needs is a place to walk and the right shoes! There is little else that needs to be done. Walking is a great way to reduce PCOS and it's a great way to get closer to nature. Mixing walking and jogging is another way to help lose some extra pounds that may be causing PCOS. It is important to walk on flat and hilly areas each time the walking is done.

Lifting weights at least two times a week is a fantastic way to burn those extra calories! Women can use personal trainers or they can do it on their own in the gym. A trainer can help to change the routine and make it easier to stay focused on losing weight and building extra muscle.

Swimming, pool aerobics, and Zumba are all immense activities for women with PCOS. The workouts that are done in the pool can help to build resistance in the body. These activities are also really easy on the joints. Stand-up paddleboarding is also a good way to build up resistance. Water sports are all grand exercises for women with PCOS.

For women who play tennis and golf, research has now shown that these are remarkable activities for those with PCOS. These sports are very challenging and with women who are trying to get more exercise and learn something new, tennis and golf are a great way to get on a new level. The cardio in tennis can help fight off the symptoms of PCOS and golf will help the leg, back, and arm muscles. Golf can also help women to focus on something other than the pain of PCOS.

Diet and exercise are important ways to resolve PCOS. Nutritionists have quite a few suggestions on what to eat when PCOS has been diagnosed. We will share some more detailed menus in order to help fight PCOS.

Nutrition for PCOS

PCOS can be caused by an unhealthy diet and even a healthy, vegetarian diet. Nutritionists have some great suggestions on the foods to eat for PCOS and the foods to avoid. These foods can help to make the symptoms go away and help women to gain their fertility and be well on their way to having a child. We have touched on the suggested foods, but we would like to share specific menus and recipes for women who have been diagnosed with PCOS.

First, we will touch on the snacks that women with PCOS can eat. When looking for snacks that are healthy and have natural sugar, fruits are generally the best idea. These include the following: apples, pears, oranges, berries, bananas, grapes, melon, kiwi, peaches, and plums. When shopping for vegetables, choose from the following: broccoli, cauliflower, tomatoes, asparagus, carrots, celery, cucumbers, eggplant, green beans, mushrooms, onions, peppers, and snap peas. Proteins are also important when planning a PCOS diet. Beans, beef, yogurt, cheese, chicken, eggs, fish, hummus, nuts, pork, tofu, and veggie burgers are all good choices. When looking at veggie burgers, look for those not made of soy and with more than nine grams of protein.

Most doctors do not suggest a lot of carbohydrates or starches with a PCOS diet, but there are some that can be eaten such as: whole wheat bread, brown rice, whole-grain cereal, corn, whole wheat English muffin, whole wheat or gluten-free pasta, sweet potatoes, and corn or whole wheat tortillas. When making dressings or prepping, these should be added to the diet: avocado, vegetable oil, corn oil, and olive oil.

Snacking can be very easy, even with PCOS. There are quite a few easy, snack ideas that those trying to reverse PCOS can enjoy. Any type of nut butter with celery, apples, or whole-wheat crackers is an easy and smart snack choice. Eating hummus with raw vegetables is another great choice for smart snacking with PCOS. If women with PCOS enjoy crackers, there are several options for them to snack on and reduced-fat cheese with crackers is one. A few other snack options are as follows: soybeans that have been dry roasted, string cheese with apples, bananas with sunflower seeds, English muffins with nut butter, low sugar yogurt with fruit or nuts in it, and Lara bars or Kind bars. When choosing these bars, it is important to look at the sugar content. Some granola bars or energy bars have large amounts of sugar in them. These bars are great for people who are constantly moving throughout the day, but for women with a slower lifestyle, the sugar can just cause weight gain and high sugar intake.

Some other snack options include hardboiled eggs, homemade trail mix with dried fruits, nuts, and dark chocolate, pomegranate seeds, low-sodium soups with beans or vegetables, single-serving pouches of tuna fish, and dark chocolate that is at least 60% cocoa. Many women with PCOS will also snack on avocados, popcorn, smoothies, chia seed pudding, and shrimp cocktail. Just because they have been diagnosed with PCOS does not mean they have to suffer when it comes to what they eat. This diet works well for many people and can benefit more than just those with PCOS.

There have been a lot of studies on the types of foods women with PCOS should be eating. There have been many rumors about how eating fruit could be bad for women with PCOS. Fruit does contain natural sugar and carbs. The sugar in fruit is not the kind of sugar in those donuts or candies. This is natural sugar that has some vitamins and minerals that table sugar does not.

Fruit is made up of entirely different types of carbs and sugars. Fructose is what it is filled with and we actually use fructose as energy. This is one of the carbs that we need in order to get through our days. The bottom line is that we need the sugar from fruits and even if women have PCOS, eating fruit is still a good idea. It does take the body a lot longer to digest the sugars in fruit though.

According to nutritionists who have patients with PCOS, it is recommended that we do eat at least two cups of fruit every day! This is what helps with good health and wellness. One serving of fruit can be considered as one small apple, one cup of grapes, one full orange, one large peach, one cup of strawberries, one cup of cherries, two small plums, and half of a large banana. Many people will add these into a smoothie and have it for breakfast in the morning. They do need to keep in mind that they need some protein in their morning smoothies too. Nuts or almond milk can be added, along with avocado to get a protein boost with the morning smoothie.

There are many myths about nutrition for women with PCOS. One of these myths is that women should go gluten-free. There is no evidence that does support this myth, but for many women with PCOS, it does help. It helps by getting them to eat fewer calories and carbs. When women spend more time trying to focus on eating more vegetables and whole grains, they can cut out the gluten if they want to. It can help them with managing their weight.

Another myth is that women should cut out dairy. There is some evidence that shows that non-fat milk can cause higher levels of androgens and insulin levels. This is why doctors will advise women to limit the amount of dairy they take in. They will suggest that the dairy they eat comes from yogurts that have probiotics in them.

Women with PCOS have noticed that it is very challenging for them to lose weight. Because PCOS does affect the insulin in the body, this could be one reason that women find losing weight difficult to do with PCOS. When they have too much insulin, there is fat storage and weight gain. This happens mostly in the midsection and this is why it is called a spare tire. Exercise is the best way to avoid fat storing in the body. If the woman is on a steady exercise plan and eating healthy, she will begin to see some changes in her weight. They may not come as quickly as she would like, but they will happen if she sticks with it.

Another reason that it is so hard for women to lose weight when they have PCOS is because of the fact that they are hungrier. Insulin also acts as an appetite stimulant. High levels of insulin mean that women will experience more hunger than usual. Women with PCOS have even reported very intense cravings that have changed their eating habits and even caused them to gain more weight. It is all right to snack, but when women snack multiple times a day, they need to make sure that they are eating foods that are healthy for them and not sugary. Protein snacks can keep women from binging on sugary and high carb foods.

PCOS can cause women to have impaired appetite-regulating hormones. This is another cause of weight loss being slower than usual. When the appetite is not regulated, women will eat and eat until they have stuffed themselves. This is not healthy and can cause them to gain weight quicker than normal. These hormones can actually stimulate hunger in the woman with PCOS instead of decreasing it. The hungrier she is, the more she will eat, and this is not healthy for women with PCOS. This makes it very difficult for women to maintain a normal weight with PCOS.

Women are encouraged to eat more fruits and vegetables when they are diagnosed with PCOS. Not eating enough fruits and vegetables can keep weight loss from happening with women with PCOS. These foods can also help women to have improvements in abdominal fat loss. Sleep apnea and other sleep disorders can also be part of the weight loss problem for women with PCOS. Sleep apnea can actually become destructive and cause weight gain in women with PCOS. Improper sleep has been one of the leading causes of obesity in women as well.

There is one medication that is said to help the symptoms of PCOS and said to help women with weight loss. This is called Victoza and many doctors have been prescribing it to their patients with PCOS. It is a medication that has been used for diabetes, but studies have shown that it can help women with PCOS. It has been helping them lose weight because it helps with the metabolism in women. It is an injectable medication that helps reduce hunger and appetite. It helps by slowing down the release of food in the stomach and making it so women want to eat less and not more. This helps them to lose weight. For women who are focused on losing more weight, they will need to ask their doctors if Victoza is perfect for them. Chances are they will be able to start it and lose that unwanted weight.

Chapter 3: Treatments for PCOS

PCOS is treatable and many doctors will suggest more natural treatments over medicine. As many women are diagnosed with it, doctors suggest these treatments because they are as simple as changing their diet and getting more exercise. Here are some more of the common natural treatments for PCOS.

One natural remedy for fighting PCOS is counting calories and being more strategic with the caloric intake in the foods that we eat. Calories have a huge impact on the glucose in the body, along with insulin and testosterone levels. When women begin to lower their insulin, they are beginning to help their infertility issues. It is amazing how much changing a diet can truly help with PCOS. There has been a lot of research done on the number of calories that women have taken in while they try to fight off PCOS. For women who ate most of their calories at breakfast time, they showed a decrease in insulin and glucose for a solid twelve weeks of watching their caloric intake. Women with PCOS who ate more calories at dinner time did not see effective results from their diet. The most effective way to diet is made up of 980 calories at breakfast, 640 calories at lunch, and 190 calories for dinner.

Another natural method of treating PCOS is by decreasing the advanced glycation end products, or AGEs, in the bloodstream. These AGEs are compounds that generally form when the glucose in the body binds with proteins, and research has shown that these AGEs contribute to causing degenerative diseases and speed up the aging process. One researcher found that by lowering the levels of AGEs in the diet can reduce levels of insulin in the body. The foods that are high in AGEs are meats, animal-derived foods, and processed foods. When these foods are grilled or roasted, the insulin levels are increased.

Taking supplements is another great way to naturally fight off PCOS. Doctors will suggest that PCOS patients take a vitamin D and calcium supplement. They also suggest taking a 1500 mg daily dose of metformin, which is a supplement being used to treat the symptoms of PCOS. Calcium and vitamin D supplements have shown vast improvements in the BMI of women with PCOS. Taking these supplements can also help to build stronger bones as women begin to age. Another suggested supplement is magnesium. When doctors see low magnesium levels in women, they are at risk for diabetes and insulin resistance. This is why taking magnesium can improve these levels and help women to fight off the symptoms of PCOS. Women who have taken these supplements have shown great changes in their insulin and glucose levels.

Chromium is one supplement that many women have never even heard of until their doctor suggested it for fighting PCOS. This is a mineral that helps to regulate the insulin and blood sugar levels in the body. Chromium helps PCOS patients to keep their blood glucose levels lower and helps them to manage their diabetes. It is important for women with PCOS to take at least 200 mcg of it daily. This will help women to fully regulate their blood sugar levels.

Eating omega-3s is another natural way to help combat the symptoms of PCOS. The omega-3s in fish can help to decrease the levels of androgens in women that have been diagnosed with PCOS. Doctors suggest that women take a least three grams of omega-3s each day for about eight or nine weeks. These studies have shown that this diet helped to lower the levels of testosterone in women's bodies. Omega-3s are found in fish, such as salmon, tuna, herring, and sardines. They are also found in nuts, seeds, flaxseed oil, soybean oil, eggs, yogurt, milk, and soy beverages.

Iron is another important mineral in the body that women with PCOS may need larger amounts of. Because many women with PCOS have heavier periods than others, they lose a lot of iron and this could cause anemia. If this is the case, doctors will suggest them taking iron supplements and eating foods higher in iron, such as spinach, eggs, and broccoli. It is important that women keep checking their iron levels because too much iron could even cause more complications of PCOS.

One thing that many women with PCOS don't want to hear is "cut out coffee". For those who drink a lot of it, doctors have suggested that it may not be the best beverage for women with PCOS. Too much caffeine can actually change the hormone levels in women and how the hormones behave in their bodies. Herbal teas are a good way to cut out coffee and kombucha can help too because of the probiotic benefits that it has. When women need the caffeine boost in the morning or mid-day, doctors suggest drinking green tea because it can help to improve insulin levels and resistance. Green tea is also a great way to manage weight loss in women with PCOS.

Eating more cinnamon can help women with PCOS too. Because cinnamon comes from cinnamon trees, it can have some positive effects on insulin levels in women with PCOS. Cinnamon is also known to help with regulating women's periods. This can help women with PCOS to have more regular periods with normal cycles. This can help to boost fertility during the times of ovulation. Turmeric is another herb that can help insulin levels in the body. It contains curcumin that can help to decrease insulin resistance and it contains anti-inflammatory benefits as well.

Evening primrose essential oil is another supplement that doctors have suggested as a natural way to fight PCOS. Evening primrose oil is often used to help women with the pain from cramps during their periods and to help with irregular periods. It can help to regulate periods and helps to improve stress levels and cholesterol levels in women. Both of these are factors for developing PCOS. Berberine is another herb that helps with insulin resistance in women with PCOS. It is used frequently in Chinese medicine and has become a popular treatment for PCOS. It can help to boost metabolism and build up the body's endocrine system.

Other Herbs for PCOS Treatments

Herbs are a very popular treatment for PCOS and there are quite a few that work very well and can help women to add some delicious new flavors into their diets. Maca root is one such herb. It comes from the maca plant and is traditionally used to help boost libido and fertility in men and women. It can also help to balance the hormone levels in women and lower cortisol levels. This is a root that can also help to treat depression that is just one of the symptoms of PCOS.

Ashwagandha is an herb that comes from India. It is a type of ginseng. It can also help to balance the cortisol levels in the body that cause depression, anxiety, and stress. With the perfect balance, women with PCOS can begin fighting off the depression they feel with PCOS. Holy basil, also known as tulsi, helps with stress levels in women as well. It can help to reduce stress, blood sugar, help with weight loss, and it has anti-inflammatory benefits. What's not to love about this herb? It also helps to lower cortisol levels.

Licorice root is an herb with similar benefits to holy basil. It is made of glycyrrhizin, which works as an anti-inflammatory and it helps balance female hormones and metabolize sugars much easier. Tribulus Terrestris is another herb that is being used to help stimulate ovulation in women with PCOS. It helps to build healthier and more regular periods as well. This herb has also been known to help to decrease the number of ovarian cysts in a woman's body.

Lastly, doctors have been suggesting the herb called chasteberry for women with PCOS. It has actually been used for hundreds of years to help with reproduction in women. It helps to relieve the symptoms of PMS and helps to boost fertility in women. There are still a lot of studies been done on it to see other benefits that it has, but women with PCOS are using it pretty regularly.

Probiotics are great for gut health and digestion. They are also being used to help treat PCOS. They do act as an anti-inflammatory and can help to regulate female sex hormones, such as estrogen and androgen. There are quite a few probiotic foods that can help boost the levels of hormones in the body. Kimchi and kombucha are two terrific examples of probiotic foods.

There are a few things to remember after being diagnosed with PCOS. Doctors may suggest herbs and supplements to take in, but they will also warn you about endocrine disruptors that should be avoided or limited. These vary from dioxins, phthalates, pesticides, BPA, and glycol ethers. These can be found in canned foods, makeup, and soaps. This is why it is always important to read labels! These endocrine disruptors can cause serious confusion when it comes to the reproductive hormones. They will try to mimic what these hormones do and that can cause an increase in PCOS symptoms.

Acupuncture is a fantastic natural way to help with the symptoms of PCOS. Acupuncture can help to boost the blood flow to the ovaries in a woman's body. It can also help to reduce cortisol levels, help with weight loss and management, and improve the body's overall sensitivity to insulin in the body. Acupuncture has been used for thousands of years in Chinese medicine and women all over the world are starting to use it to help them fight off the symptoms of PCOS.

There are many types of natural treatments for PCOS. Doctors may suggest these before they suggest medications, but it is important to remember that all women's bodies are different and some of these supplements will work differently on each person. If a woman tries all of these natural treatments and has no luck with them, it is important that she goes to her doctor. Her doctor will be able to explain different treatments that are on the market today and how they can change her body. There are treatments to be aware of such as progestin, which makes it very tough for women to get pregnant. Systemic enzyme therapies and supplements that say they cure instantly are both two treatments to be wary of. These treatments may not work on women with PCOS and can disrupt any chances a woman has in getting pregnant. This is why it is always important to turn to medical doctors for their professional opinions on how to fight PCOS.

Medical Treatments for PCOS

Even though there are many natural treatments for PCOS, doctors have also recommenced quite a few medical treatments that do involve prescription drugs. The medications that doctors prescribe all have helpful benefits for women who are suffering from PCOS. Women may have to try several types of medications before they find the one that works best for them.

Clomiphene, also known as Clomid, is one medication that doctors have suggested women use to help fight off PCOS. Women who are having problems becoming pregnant generally use Clomid. It helps the body stimulate an increase in hormones. These hormones help the growth and release of an egg during ovulation. Women with PCOS may have problems with releasing their eggs during ovulation and this can cause infertility in them.

Clomid does have some side effects that women need to be aware of. It can cause upset stomach, bloating, hot flashes, tenderness in the breasts, and dizziness. When experiencing any of these side effects, it's important for women to always tell their doctor. Some medications do not work well with a woman's body, so it is always a good idea to be upfront with their doctor.

Another medication that doctors suggest for PCOS is Letrozole, or Femara. This medication was introduced as a way to treat breast cancer in women if they are diagnosed after menopause. It is also being used as a way to treat PCOS. It helps to decrease the estrogen amounts in the body. The side effects that it can have are hot flashes, muscle pains, sweating, and insomnia.

Metformin is another type of medication that is suggested for PCOS patients. It helps to improve the insulin levels in the body and insulin resistance. Doctors who have patients who are also on a diet and fitness program to help with their PCOS and blood sugar levels suggest this drug. It is mainly used by patients with type 2 diabetes but has become a great medication for PCOS symptoms. It can help regulate blood sugar and help to prevent sexual function problems. It can restore the response to insulin by the body and decrease the amount of sugar in the liver. The side effects of this medication are vomiting, dizziness, and an upset stomach.

Gonadotrophins can also be used to help regulate the hormones in the body. These are a type of fertility medication that is injected into a woman. They are generally used as a fertility drug. They can begin at the beginning of the menstrual cycle in order to help many eggs grow in size. The more eggs grow to be mature in size, the more likely a woman will get pregnant. This helps PCOS because it can help women with ovulating.

Birth control pills are also used to help combat PCOS. They are used to help regulate a woman's period and this is a way to make it more predictable and easier for a woman to determine if she is able to get pregnant. Birth control can help PCOS in quite a few ways and that is why doctors have started to prescribe it to fight off symptoms. The pills help to regulate different hormone imbalances too. A woman can increase her estrogen levels and lower the testosterone levels when she takes birth control pills regularly.

Not all women can take birth control pills in order to fight off PCOS. There are risks to some women such as a higher risk of diabetes. Women who have heart issues may not be able to take birth control either. There are side effects from them that can cause blood clots in the body. Women that have PCOS and are obese have a much higher risk of developing these issues. Weight gain is another side effect of birth control pills and women who have weight problems already may not be the best candidates for them. Gaining this extra weight can actually make PCOS symptoms much worse.

Birth control pills all work to help the female hormones become much more balanced. These pills help the period to be regulated and keep women from having a child until they decide that they want one. They can also help with the cervix as well. Birth control pills thicken the mucus there. When women take birth control, they will still release their eggs during ovulation, but the thicker cervix mucus will help them from getting pregnant while on the pill. There are many brands of the birth control pill and they include:

Aviane, Estrostep, Lessina, Loestrin, Nordette, Ortho-Novum, Yasmin, and Yaz to name a few. Loestrin has lower levels of estrogen in it and those can help with the symptoms of PCOS.

Reducing Other PCOS Symptoms with Medications

Hair growth and loss are two symptoms of PCOS. Doctors have recommended many types of medication to help this. One of those is Aldactone. This medication helps to block the effects that androgen has on the skin. It can also be used to treat high blood pressure and heart problems. It is known to help prevent strokes and kidney problems. This drug has some intense side effects though. It is not to be taken while trying to conceive a child because it can cause birth defects in children. When doctors suggest using this pill to combat PCOS, they make sure that their patients are on birth control first.

Another product that doctors suggest for hair growth in women is Vaniqa. As women begin to age, hormones change. When women are diagnosed with PCOS, the hormone changes can cause extreme hair growth on their faces. This is a cream that can actually slow down the hair growth in women. This cream works best when it is used on the face and under the chin. This cream is only for the face and it can actually block hormones that cause the hairs to come up on the face. It helps to slow down the growth and to make the hairs on the face lighter in color and fine. This cream can cause burning of the skin, so it is important that patients test it out first in order to be sure they do not have an allergic reaction to it.

When women are diagnosed with PCOS, their chances of developing type 2 diabetes can also increase. This is why doctors will suggest using medications that help with diabetes. One of these medications is called Glucophage. This drug can help reduce the insulin resistance in a woman and can also improve the regularity of a woman's cycle.

Hormone medication can also be helpful to a woman when she is diagnosed with PCOS. These hormones vary but can help with infertility and other symptoms of PCOS. Follicle-stimulating hormones are being used to help a woman to stimulate the growth of her eggs. This can help her to become pregnant quicker and help with a healthy pregnancy. Luteinizing hormone can help with the release of the eggs from the ovaries. This is another hormone recommended for women with PCOS.

Doctors have also recommended hormones such as human chorionic gonadotrophin, which helps to make the egg reach maturity so a woman can have a baby,

Estrace that prepared the woman's uterus to receive an egg, and Provera that helps the uterus get ready for implantation of the egg. There are plenty of these hormones that women with PCOS can take in order to become pregnant. Menopur and Bravelle are two more of the hormones that can help women with PCOS. There are supplements that women can take for PCOS that are non-hormonal. These supplements can also help to increase the chances of pregnancy in women with PCOS.

Women have many options when it comes to fighting PCOS. With natural remedies and prescribed medications, women with PCOS who want to become pregnant, do have a chance at doing so.

Chapter 4: Getting Pregnant with PCOS

PCOS affects over five million women in the world. One of the most common symptoms is infertility. Women who are diagnosed with PCOS may think that there is no way for them to become pregnant, but that is not the truth. There are actually ways to get pregnant, even with PCOS. There are fertility hormones that can help and medications, which we previously mentioned. There are many other ways to become pregnant with PCOS as well.

One common symptom of PCOS is weight gain and obesity. Losing weight is an easy way to help restart ovulation. Women who are obese and have PCOS do not ovulate regularly and this can cause big problems with infertility. Women with PCOS may experience what is called severe anovulation. Severe anovulation occurs when women have irregular periods. This can also lead to abnormal levels of progesterone, thicker endometrium, and lack of cervical mucus. Women with this dysfunction will miss their periods often and some of these women may never get a period. The cycles of these women will last about 20 days, but sometimes shorter. This causes ovulation to be dysfunctional and can cause infertility. Anovulation can be caused by obesity, but there are other causes. Low body weight, extreme exercise, ovarian failure, thyroid issues, and high levels of stress can all cause this dysfunction in women.

Research has shown that when women lose the extra weight that they have put on, they are helping in the restarting ovulation process. Women only have to lose about five to ten percent of the extra weight that they have recently added on. Losing this weight will help to push the menstrual cycle and help get it back to normal. This won't happen instantly though. When women work hard with diet and exercise, they will begin to see some changes in their weight and with their menstrual cycles. There has not been any evidence that shows that being thinner helps to conceive a child and some women do find that they need fertility drugs in order to do so.

One of the easiest diets to follow when diagnosed with PCOS is a low-carb diet. A low-carb diet consists of eating foods that are rich in nutrients and low in sugar. Junk food is one of the worst things that women with PCOS can eat and this is another way to pack on the pounds. Here are some food suggestions for a low-carb diet:

- Lean meat: chicken breasts, pork, and sirloin

- Fish

- Eggs
- Leafy greens
- Broccoli
- Cauliflower
- Seeds and Nuts
- Nut Butter
- Coconut oil
- Olive Oil
- Apples
- Blueberries
- Strawberries
- Plain Greek yogurt

When on a low-carb diet, it is important that women know exactly much of the carbs they are taking in. Most of the low-carb diets on the market today allow just about twenty to forty grams of carbs per day. When looking at items like bread or pasta, we can see that they both contain well over the daily suggested amount. This is why it is key to cut out the carbs when diagnosed with PCOS.

Low-carb diets may be difficult to start at first, but there are easy ways to manage them. Making a meal plan is an easy way to get a low-carb diet, or any other type of diet started. This doesn't take too much time to do and when it is all written out, shopping for the week can be a breeze. Making a meal plan is a great idea because it will help women stick to it. With the full list in their hand each time they go shopping, they will have something to follow and never have to stray from the list. There are many websites that can even help women write up recipe ideas and help to make shopping easier. Going on a diet doesn't mean that they give up the foods they love, they will just have to try eating them in new ways.

When a meal plan is made, this will help to avoid the unhealthy choices at the grocery store. The only problem with making a meal plan is that there may be a change of plans in the week. Sometimes they will go out to eat with their partner or colleagues. This makes it tough to follow the diet, but they can look through the menu about the different options they have. This doesn't have to be complicated, it's just important to not eat fast food or foods high in carbs and sugars.

Meal planning is very easy to do and when the shopping has been done, meal prep is the next step when following a low-carb diet. Preparing meals can be very easy and when all of this is done at the beginning of the week, there is nothing to worry about when packing lunches each morning. Planning and prepping help to avoid making the unhealthy food choices, save a lot of time, save a lot of money, and make it worth it when there is extra time in the morning to catch up on other chores. Meal prep can be as easy as packing and freezing the meals for the week.

There are many great choices for low-carb snacks too. Hard-boiled eggs, unsweetened yogurt, carrots, nuts, cheese, and nut butter are all a great snack to eat during the day. It is easy to find healthy snacks for those times in between meals and snacking does help to avoid eating too much at mealtimes.

Dieting and exercise are just two of the ways to help to restart the ovulation cycle. Once women begin to lose weight, they will start to notice some changes. Their chances of diabetes will be lowered and they will begin to have more energy. Their self-esteem will also grow because of losing the unwanted pounds they have. When they begin to watch the foods that they are eating, they will have more vitamins and nutrients in their lives too. This will help them to work on a healthier lifestyle.

Diets for Boosting Fertility

Women with PCOS who are obese may have a tough time losing weight. The great thing is that there are actually different types of diets that can boost fertility, with or without PCOS. The first of these is a Mediterranean style diet. This is a diet that includes more plant-based foods. The focus on this type of diet are foods like nuts, seeds, fruits, vegetables, and beans. Those who follow this diet eat up to six servings of fruits and vegetables each day! This diet also includes eating seafood or fish twice a week. This diet uses olive oil for cooking instead of butter.

The Mediterranean diet has some healthy options when it comes to eating meat too. The choices for this diet are chicken and eggs. They eat the meat more like it is a side dish and the vegetables are the entree. They do eat low sugar yogurt and cheeses as well. There are very few red meat dishes and sweets in this diet.

Another diet that can help improve fertility in women is the Nurses' Health fertility diet. In this diet, there is a lot of exercise incorporated into healthy eating patterns. This diet includes eating more foods like avocado, lentils and beans, oatmeal, wheat bread, foods high in fiber and iron, and multivitamins. This diet concentrates more on having a healthy weight and doing regular exercise.

There is another diet that can help fertility because it helps with insulin resistance. Women with PCOS do have a tendency to have issues with their insulin levels and this diet can help. This diet includes food that is low glycemic, eating more complex carbs, getting more calories from proteins such as eggs, fish, and meat, eating a big breakfast and smaller dinners. This diet also incorporates more exercise and pairing foods that can help insulin levels in the body.

Women with PCOS have been very curious about having a vegan diet and if it can be healthy while getting pregnant and while pregnant. A vegan diet is actually very healthy for women with PCOS and for those who are trying to become pregnant. There may be some nutrient deficiencies, but it is easy to find supplements for these nutrients. It is important that when trying to get pregnant and eating a vegan diet, women continue to have regular doctor visits in order to keep an eye on their health. A vegan diet means that the followers of it do not eat anything that comes from animals. They do not eat eggs, milk, cheese, etc. Vegan women who are trying to get pregnant will have to follow a close diet where they can find foods to supplement the nutrients that they are not getting from their diet.

Vegan diets have not shown to cause any complications in pregnancy, which is very good news.

This diet could cause anemia in those who follow it, but iron supplements are a great way to add to the diet. Because of the diet, it is important that women who follow the vegan diet get enough B-12 in their diets. Most B-12 does come from eggs and milk, so getting it from other sources is important since vegans do not include these in their diets. For women who follow a vegan diet, it is key to get enough dark leafy greens, asparagus, broccoli, beans, and lentils. These foods have a lot of B 12 and folate in them that can help with a healthier birth and baby. There are also prenatal vitamins that women can take that can help boost these nutrients.

Anemia is another problem that women who eat vegan may have. This is a lack of iron in the body. This is a big concern for women who are vegans and pregnant. There is not a lot of iron in a plant-based diet, but there are ways to get the extra iron in foods in the vegan diet. These foods include:

- Beans
- Lentils
- Nuts
- Seeds
- Dried fruit

- Leafy Greens
- Quinoa
- Molasses
- Peanut Butter
- Brown rice
- Tofu

Getting enough vitamin C is also important for women who eat vegan. There are many foods that they can still enjoy and stay with their diet. These foods are high in vitamin C and include:

- Orange juice
- Pineapple
- Strawberries
- Kiwi
- Brussels Sprouts
- Yellow Bell Peppers

When eating a vegan diet, there are a lot of foods that women can still eat and get the vitamins and nutrients that they need. Some doctors will suggest other supplements in order to make sure the woman and baby are healthy throughout the entire pregnancy. Protein is one of these nutrients that many vegans need help getting. Protein comes from beans and whole grains. A pregnant woman needs to get at least 100 grams of protein each day. This is why it can be difficult for women who are vegan. There are gluten-free pastas that are full of protein, along with beans and lentils.

Vitamin D is also important for a healthy pregnancy. This can come from milk alternatives and leafy greens. Many doctors will put their vegan patients on vitamin D supplements. Calcium is another important nutrient that many vegan women get low numbers of. There are many foods that are rich in calcium though. These foods include:

- Almond milk
- Pinto beans
- Red beans
- White beans
- Bok choy
- Kale

- Spinach

- Broccoli

- Sweet potatoes

A vegan diet may sound like a great way to lose weight and maintain a healthy life. There are some types of vegan diets that can be unhealthy though. Many vegans find it hard to get enough calories and for women with PCOS, this could cause an unhealthy pregnancy. A vegan diet that is high in carbs is not the best one to follow. Too many carbs per day can cause some weight gain and cause an unhealthy pregnancy. This could also make PCOS symptoms worse. Vegans must pay very close attention to their diets. Once they have their vitamin and nutrient levels balanced, they can rest assured that they will be able to have a healthy pregnancy and their fertility rates will be much better.

One diet that has been said to cause a lot of fertility is problems is called the Western Diet. This diet has been shown to cause obesity and diabetes. The foods in this diet are to be avoided at all costs, especially for women who have been diagnosed with PCOS. We simply want to show women what not to eat and why it could be destroying their body. This diet includes red meat and processed meats, white bread, pizza, snacks, energy drinks, and sweets. This diet has caused fertility problems in men and damaged their sperm counts. Doctors countered this diet with one called the Prudent Diet that includes more fish and chicken, fruits and vegetables, beans, and whole grains. Men who switched diets showed a better sperm count and their sperm were going in the right direction during intercourse.

Fertility Foods

These diets may all have special nutrients and vitamins that can help to increase fertility in women. There are specific foods that can also help to boost fertility. These foods include sunflower seeds and sunflower seed butter. These seeds may boost fertility because they are a great source of vitamin E. Vitamin E has been shown to boost fertility in men and women. It is also high in folate, selenium, and zinc. Sunflower seeds also have a large amount of omega 3 and 6. There are ways to get more sunflower seeds in the diet too. They can be sprinkled on salads, used on sandwiches, used in smoothies, and just eaten as a snack.

Fruits have some great nutrients that can also help to increase fertility. Grapefruit and orange juice can help to boost fertility by being extremely high in putrescine. This is a hormone that can help improve the health of eggs in women. These juices both have large amounts of vitamin C in them as well. Vitamin C can help to boost the hormone balance in women and this can help to aid in fertility. Women can make smoothies with these juices or add the fruit to salads.

There has been some research done that eating older cheeses can actually help with fertility. Cheeses such as cheddar, Parmesan, and Manchego have high amounts of polyamines in them. These are proteins that can help the reproductive system. They can help to improve sperm count and help women to improve their egg health. This can help them to become pregnant much easier. It is important to watch the amount of cheese taken in because it does contain a lot of fat and calories. It can help with fertility issues though.

What if someone told you that ice cream could help fertility? Well, it can! Foods such as sherbet, yogurt, cottage cheese, whole milk, ice cream, and cream cheese can all help with boosting fertility. These foods help women that have shown fertility problems in the past and problems with ovulation. Just like with mature cheeses, it is important to watch the intake of these foods. They do have the potential to help women pack on a few more pounds, which leads to obesity. This is why it's a good idea to not overdo it with these foods.

Cow liver is another food that has been shown to help with fertility problems. Cow liver has quite a long list of nutrients in it and many of them help with reproductive health in men and women. Cow liver contains vitamin A, vitamin B12, riboflavin, folate, selenium, choline, zinc, and coenzyme Q10. These vitamins and minerals help to boost the health of female eggs, semen health, reduce the risk of birth defects, and help to boost regular menstruation in women.

Cooked tomatoes are another great food for fertility. Cooked tomatoes can be found in soups or can be cooked on the grill or oven. They are high in antioxidants such as lycopene. This is a very important antioxidant for men and women. It helps to treat infertility in both. These cooked tomatoes have also helped women to become pregnant after eating them for about a year. Lentils and beans are another group of foods that have astonishing results in helping fertility problems. Black beans are one of the best actually. These beans are a great source of protein and help with ovulation problems. Lentils have high quantities of polyamine spermidine. This can help to better fertilize an egg. They are also a source of folate that can help with healthier embryos.

Asparagus may smell funny, but it is another healthy source for helping with fertility. Cooked asparagus contains folate, vitamin K, zinc, selenium, vitamin A, vitamin, C, and thiamin. These nutrients help to boost the fertility of men and women. There are so many great ways to cook asparagus and it is very good for the body too!

Another food that can help to boost fertility is oysters. Slippery and slimy, they have many benefits that can help women to increase their fertility. Not only are oysters very low in calories, but they also contain many nutrients and vitamins. They contain almost 50% of the daily iron needed per day, vitamin B-12, selenium, and zinc. In fact, they contain almost 200% of the daily zinc needed daily! Raw is the best way to eat oysters and they can help to give women healthier eggs and boost the sperm count in men. They are also used as a natural aphrodisiac.

Pomegranates are a delicious choice when it comes to eating foods for fertility. They are high in antioxidants that can help to boost fertility in men and women. The juice in pomegranates can help to increase the sperm count in men. Walnuts are another food known to help reproduction in men and women. The amount of omega 3 and 6 in walnuts is part of the reason that they help to boost reproductive hormones. Walnuts can also help to improve the health of semen.

Eating eggs is another way to boost fertility. Eggs have quite a bit of B vitamins and omega 3. The lean protein in eggs helps to boost fertility in both men and women. They also contain choline that helps to reduce the risk of birth defects in children. Pineapple is a very sweet and healthy treat that can help fertility problems. Pineapple has been said to be a great food to eat when trying to have a baby. It is a very good source of vitamin C and women with PCOS need the extra boost of vitamin C whenever they can get it. Pineapple can also boost sperm counts in men. Pineapple also contains bromelain, which has anti-inflammatory benefits.

Many doctors recommend their PCOS patients eat more fish and they have the right idea about this! Fish contains omega 3's that can really help to boost fertility. Salmon is one of the best to eat! Salmon is a great food for many health ailments and fertility is on the top of that list. When trying to get pregnant, women should be eating wild-caught salmon in order to keep the mercury levels down. Salmon also contains fatty acids that can help to boost sperm counts in men and healthy eggs in women. Salmon also contains vitamin D and selenium. In fact, salmon gives us about 97% of the daily dosage of vitamin D.

Many people wouldn't think that cinnamon can help boost fertility, but it has a lot of health benefits. Because PCOS is associated with insulin resistance, doctors suggest eating more cinnamon. Cinnamon can help to improve the health of those who have diabetes and it can also help to fight it off. Women who eat more cinnamon have shown some great ovulation improvements and their periods have become much more regular. Cinnamon is easy to add to the diet too. Just a sprinkle of cinnamon in the tea, coffee, oatmeal, or yogurt can help so much! It is not only very helpful, but it is also delicious. It is one of the herbs that should be added into anyone's diet no matter what!

All of these foods have great health benefits and fertility-boosting benefits. Once women with PCOS start to eat more of them, they will begin to see health changes and ovulation and menstruation changes. There are several ways that they can maintain a healthy diet and these foods will point them in the right direction too!

Gluten-Free for Fertility

Researchers have been doing studies about the effects of gluten and infertility. Gluten is now being blamed for quite a few ailments and now infertility is one of them! Celiac disease is just one autoimmune disease that is caused by eating too much gluten. It causes a lot of horrible changes in health. Many people who have it don't know that they do and it will go misdiagnosed. Women who are diagnosed with it may be at risk for infertility issues. In fact, women that have recently reported having miscarriages may have celiac disease. When it does go undiagnosed, celiac disease can cause miscarriages and irregular periods.

Many women have noticed that as soon as they began a gluten-free diet, their bodies began to change for the best. They noticed that their periods had become regular and they were able to conceive a child naturally and without fertility drugs. Changing the diet can help women in so many ways and cutting out gluten is just one. There are other types of gluten sensitivities that are not caused by celiac disease though.

Women with PCOS who have an intolerance to gluten, but do not have Celiac disease could be suffering from something else. If the allergy has shown itself to the women, it is important that they listen to their body and stop eating gluten. Non-celiac sensitivity is part of a condition that actually has many other symptoms. Those who suffer from it will show the exact same signs a Celiac disease, but it may be a bit smaller. Gluten allergies can cause problems in the intestines, so it is important for women to get this under control. When these gluten allergies are not treated, there can be fertility problems that arise.

Inflammatory bowel disease and Crohn's disease can both cause problems with fertility if they are not treated in the proper ways. Crohn's can cause miscarriages and infertility. When diagnosed with these, it is important that women take all of the right steps in order to change their diets and lifestyle, especially if getting pregnant is what they want to do in the future.

PCOS diets recommend cutting out carbs and reducing the amount of gluten. Foods that are high in gluten can cause problems with insulin resistance and blood sugar levels. There hasn't been proof that gluten and PCOS can cause problems with fertility, but gluten is shown to be a problem with diabetics. Cutting down on the gluten in the diet is one of the best ways to reduce the chances of getting diabetes and helping to keep the blood sugar balanced.

Going gluten-free can be done and in a very healthy way. When women with PCOS are trying to conceive, their doctors will suggest changing the diet first and cutting out the gluten could be just one of the ways to do so. The research is still being done on the connection but making a diet healthier and with less gluten never hurt anyone!

Vitamin Supplements for Pregnancy

PCOS can cause many vitamin and nutrient deficiencies. This can cause problems such as infertility and unhealthy pregnancies. This is why doctors will recommend supplements to their patients with PCOS. B vitamins are very important when it comes to fertility and fighting off the symptoms of PCOS. B vitamins help to fight off anemia and keep the red blood cells working properly. B vitamins for fertility are generally B-6 and B-9. B-9 contains large amounts of folate, which we have seen be very important in the fertility and pregnancy process. Low levels of B-9 can also be a factor in irregular periods in women.

Vitamin C is another vitamin that women with PCOS may not get quite enough of. Vitamin C helps to keep our immune systems strong and healthy. When women with PCOS have lower levels of it, it can cause medical risks for them, especially when they want to get pregnant. Vitamin C also works as a very strong antioxidant. Antioxidants are fantastic at helping women to get pregnant and help to boost their fertility. Free radicals attack our bodies as we age and in women, they can do damage to the body in ways that will lower fertility. This is why taking vitamin C supplements can help greatly!

There is one nutrient that we have yet to touch on and it is coenzyme Q10. Q10 is another potent antioxidant that helps with fertility in women. It can also help men's sperm counts and motility in the sperm. Women who are thinking of doing in vitro fertilization have had higher results when their levels of Q10 was higher. Very low levels of vitamin D are often associated with infertility too. The more vitamin D a woman has in her body, the higher her chances are for getting pregnant and having regular ovulation cycles. High levels of vitamin D also can help cut the risk of endometriosis.

Selenium is something that we have talked about quite a bit in this book so far. It is important for fertility and in women who are trying to become pregnant. Selenium also can help with thyroid functions and lowering stress levels, both are incredibly important when it is time to conceive and carry a child. Adding selenium to the diet can help a woman to boost her fertility and it can also help with men's sperm health.

There are large numbers of fertility vitamins and supplements found online. It is important that a doctor is consulted before trying any of these supplements. The online stores will make promises that these are the best, all-natural ways to conceive, but it is always a good option to do the research. We have made a complete list of the vitamins and supplements that will help fertility. Here are the following vitamins for fertility:

- Folate
- Zinc
- B-vitamins

- Vitamin C

- Vitamin E

- Magnesium

- Selenium

Many vitamins do contain antioxidants and there are several foods and drinks where antioxidants come from. Green tea is a great source of antioxidants. It also has some very positive effects on sperm counts in men.

Amino acids are essential for women and men to conceive a child. The human body does make amino acids, but we can also get them from the foods we eat. Amino acids that come to us from foods are L-arginine and L-carnitine. These amino acids help to get the blood flowing to the uterus and the ovaries. They can also help to keep the eggs healthy in the female body.

When searching online for fertility supplements, one that may come up is chaste tree berry. This is sometimes called vitex. This is a supplement that women can use for boosting their fertility and staying healthy. It helps to improve ovulation and regulate menstrual cycles. DHEA is another supplement that is all over the health world. It is a hormone that we already have in our bodies. It helps to boost ovarian health. It can be purchased online and many women choose it in order to combat PCOS symptoms. It can raise androgen levels in women, but it can also have some side effects, such as hair growth and irregular periods.

Be careful when it comes to buying fertility supplements online. Always check in with a doctor first to find out how effective they really are. A lot of these products will make promises to their customers, but they are not always true. The products that say they are the best and they can help women get pregnant no matter what, probably are not the best ones to buy. No supplement can guarantee that a woman gets pregnant and it cannot cure infertility either. There are supplements that will say "doctors choose this", but they never list a name of these doctors. If the product cannot follow up with proper evidence, then it probably won't help boost fertility.

Bad Habits and Fertility

We have talked about many ways to boost fertility in the form of diets, exercises, and supplements. There are so many bad habits that men and women have that can also be the major factor in infertility problems. One of these is staying up too late and losing valuable sleep. Bad sleeping habits can actually cause irregular periods. There is also a very small number of women who suffered from miscarriages. The women in this study worked the night shifts at hospitals and bars. Poor sleep also can lead to weight problems. Like we have mentioned earlier, weight problems can lead to infertility and other reproductive issues. Getting a good night's sleep can change all of these issues and once the body is on a schedule, everything will begin to feel better.

Caffeine is another bad habit that many of us need to break. Too much caffeine can actually cause problems with fertility. We all love our coffee and tea in the morning, but if women are drinking over 300 mg per day, they may have lower chances of getting pregnant and being able to maintain a healthy pregnancy. The risk of miscarriages can be much greater if there is too much caffeine in the system as well. More than two cups of coffee are about 300 mg or six cups of tea. Drinking too much coffee can also be a cause for bad sleep at night, so cutting out the caffeine could be one way to solve two bad habits!

Overeating and having poor eating habits are two other bad habits that could cause infertility. Binging on food that isn't healthy can cause obesity and weight gain can change the reproductive health of women. Junk food can cause problems with blood sugar and can cause diabetes. There is a connection between fertility and insulin levels and this is why we have made it clear that eating healthy is better for the body and reproductive health.

Drinking too much alcohol is another bad habit that can cause fertility problems in men and women. Occasional drinks are completely fine for the body, but when the drinking becomes a problem, there are issues that fertility will face. Men who drink a lot have unhealthy sperm counts. Women who drink more than three drinks a week may face the problem of not being able to get pregnant right away. Drinking is fun to do and we all do it to celebrate, but when it becomes a problem, it is time to choose between reproductive health and too much fun.

Not only is smoking a horrible habit to have, but it can also cause fertility problems. Smoking can cause problems in the fallopian tubes that can cause an ectopic pregnancy. The risk of cervical cancer increases for women who smoke as well. Women who smoke may also have damage in the ovaries and their reproductive health may not be the best for having a child. Secondhand smoke can also have a huge impact on fertility. Women who have partner's that smoke have more of a chance of reducing their fertility levels.

For women who engage in unsafe sex, there is a chance of contracting STDs. These STDs are one of the only known cases of infertility that are completely preventable. STDs such as gonorrhea and chlamydia can cause pelvic inflammatory disease if they are not treated right away. This can cause women to be infertile and it will eventually block the fallopian tubes. STDs such as herpes and syphilis can cause miscarriages and even infant deaths.

By looking at all of these changes that we can make to our lives, we hope that PCOS is easier to fight off. Women with PCOS need all of the help that they can get when it comes to conceiving a child in a healthy manner. By breaking bad habits, eating right, and getting all of the vitamins and minerals that they need, they will improve their chances of getting pregnant quicker than usual.

Chapter 5: Menopause and PCOS

Although many women are diagnosed with PCOS during the time of their lives when they are still able to conceive children, there are many women who are diagnosed with it during menopause. For women who have PCOS and they just entered menopause, there may be a lot of changes happening in the reproductive organs added onto the hot flashes and mood swings that they have to deal with as well. The average age for starting menopause is around 51, but some women will experience it earlier or even later. There are women who naturally began menopause at the age of 40 and some that have had it start as late as 61 years old! Menopause begins when a woman has not had a regular period for over a year, or twelve consecutive months. Menopause will last anywhere from two to eight years. Many women will get through this change much quicker than others.

When menopause hits, there are many changes that a woman's body will go through. A woman will begin to notice changes in her periods. Sometimes the periods are lighter than ever, while at other times, they are heavy and very painful. The time between periods will change as well and a woman may see months between her periods until they stop coming completely. For some women, they may have irregular periods years before menopause has even started. This is why menopause can get very frustrating and trying to figure out if it has started is difficult to do at times. All cases of women are different and the way the body changes is never the same in anyone.

Menopause has quite a few symptoms that women dread as they grow older. One of these is hot flashes. Hot flashes are the most common sign that menopause has begun. A hot flash is simply a warm feeling that comes on in the face or neck area. These hot flashes are very intense and some women will wake up covered in sweat from having them late at night when they are sleeping. Hot flashes don't actually last very long. They will generally last anywhere from ten to thirty seconds each time they come on.

Sleeping issues are another symptom of menopause. Insomnia can be caused by the hot flashes and changes in hormones can also cause issues with sleeping patterns at night. Sexual problems also stem from menopause. With so many changes occurring in the body, women's hormones can change greatly during menopause. Some women will notice that their intercourse has become very painful from the lack of moisture in the vagina. There are also changes in the libido that occur during menopause. Some women notice that their libido was going crazy! They couldn't have enough sex with their partner, while others have no interest in sex whatsoever when they hit menopause. For women who can't get enough sex during menopause, it is important to practice birth control. There are many babies born to women who are in menopause. It is possible to have a baby during the change of life.

The hormones that are affected by PCOS include testosterone and progesterone. When menopause is beginning, these hormones may already be dropping. As they age, women will make less estrogen and progesterone and this will cause them to stop ovulating eventually. PCOS can cause problems with hormones and the blood, but in different ways when a woman is going through menopause. This is why doctors have said that going through menopause does not help to cure PCOS. Many women aren't sure if they have PCOS or they are going into perimenopause. Perimenopause begins right before menopause does. There are many symptoms to it such as hot flashes and periods that are irregular. Hormones will begin to change and the body may start to go in different directions. Perimenopause can actually last a few years and leads the way to menopause.

The symptoms of PCOS and perimenopause are similar in many ways such as infertility, mood swings, sleeping troubles, thinning hair, unwanted hair growth, weight gain, and skin and acne problems. PCOS is completely manageable when a woman is in perimenopause. Weight control is one of the biggest factors in helping to fight off PCOS and other health problems. As female hormones change, their weight may be the first noticeable change in their body. Being overweight for a woman can increase other health problems, such as heart attacks and diabetes. Managing the weight is key to do during perimenopause and with PCOS. Getting a better night's sleep is also key when it comes to fighting off perimenopause symptoms and PCOS symptoms.

Will PCOS and menopause actually affect the other? Yes is the short answer to this question. As we have explained, there are many changes that do occur in a woman's body with PCOS and during menopause. The two will end up working hand in hand at some point on a woman's body. With women who have PCOS, they have noticed that they will go through menopause one to two years later than women that do not have PCOS. This could have something to do with the role that the hormones play in women with PCOS. PCOS gives women an unbalanced set of hormones and this could be one of the reasons that menopause affects it.

PCOS and menopause are very similar to the other. During both of them, women may experience missing their periods, infertility, mood changes, problems sleeping, and weight gain. PCOS is different in some ways because it can cause headaches, pain in the pelvic area, and terrible skin problems. In PCOS, there are no reported signs of libido changes, whereas, menopause brings on some drastic changes in libido. When women do notice these changes occurring, there are actually things that they can do to help themselves to feel better.

Managing weight is key during menopause and with PCOS. Obesity can cause many health problems so a balanced diet and exercise are two easy ways to lose weight. We have given many options on diets and eating right to help lose weight when diagnosed with PCOS. These tips work well during menopause as well. As of now, there is no known cure for PCOS, but there are ways to combat the symptoms. Menopause will only last a couple of years and there are ways to get through that as well. If women are aware of the changes that are occurring in their bodies, they will be ready for the next step in their lives. PCOS doesn't have to stop them from enjoying life or from getting through menopause.

Some women have brought up questions about PCOS getting better if they have a hysterectomy. It is not yet proven that having a hysterectomy can help to cure PCOS. Many women think that because PCOS is in the ovaries that changing them could get rid of it.

That is not the case though. Hysterectomies are not always the answer for women who are having ovarian problems. There are many women, about 600,000 or so that have hysterectomies each year. This is not an easy surgery. In fact, it is invasive and painful for any woman who has it. It is the removal of the ovaries and fallopian tubes. There are types of hysterectomies where the uterus is removed as well. The cervix will remain place though. These surgeries take at least six months for a woman to recover from. That is why many doctors suggest the surgery only if it is needed for the woman to be healthier.

There are cases of women having hysterectomies to prevent pregnancy or to help them with their periods. They are only suggested if a woman suffers from heavy periods that last for weeks and cause intense bleeding and pain, fibroids, severe pelvic pain, severe endometriosis, and cancer in the reproductive organs.

Hysterectomies do cause a woman to go into early menopause. This will completely stop the periods and hormone levels will begin to drop. There are many problems that happen as soon as a woman has a hysterectomy. These problems vary from vaginal dryness, low libido, insomnia, urinary incontinence, and a great risk of osteoporosis.

Why does the hysterectomy not cure PCOS? Women will still produce androgens after the surgery. Because there are no ovaries, women will still experience the elevated levels of androgens. The adrenal glands will still produce testosterone and they may try to make more because the ovaries are no longer in the body to produce estrogen. This is when women begin to suffer from excessive hair growth on their bodies. A hysterectomy doesn't cure PCOS because women will still have metabolic problems. A woman's weight will still need to be managed and chances for heart disease and diabetes may actually rise after the surgery. When hormones are going crazy, chances are a woman is eating more than she should. This calls for a diet that is rich in vitamins, nutrients, and antioxidants.

Hysterectomies are not a surgery that doctors will suggest unless it is absolutely needed. There are many physical side effects that can cause emotional stress in women. Once the surgery is complete, a woman will need to stay in the hospital for anywhere from one to three days. There will be some blood that is discharged from the body and there may even be cramps that will feel like menstrual cramps. This is completely normal after the surgery.

Some women will recover quicker than others, but it depends on the woman's body and tolerance to pain.

Many women will return to their normal activities about six weeks after their surgery. Some will only take three to four weeks to recover. After a hysterectomy, women may notice the following:

- pain at the incision area

- swelling and bruising at the incision area

- burning and itching at the incision area

- numbness near the incision area and down the leg

- hot flashes

- vaginal dryness

- night sweats

- insomnia

Emotions are another part of the side effects of having a hysterectomy. Because the uterus has been taken out of the body, women may begin to feel that they are missing a part of themselves. This is completely normal after a surgery like this one. This can be a difficult change for a woman and this is what causes her emotions to go crazy! Some women are relieved after they have the surgery, while those who wanted to have a child may feel saddened by their loss. Women all respond differently mainly because of the reasoning behind having the surgery.

There are long term side effects of having a hysterectomy as well. Some women have suffered from pelvic organ prolapse and had to have surgery to correct it. Sometimes the vagina can bulge outside of the body after this surgery. This is because it is no longer connected to the cervix and uterus. This is a major change that happens in many women who have had a hysterectomy. Some of the other organs can change as well. The bowels and bladder may push on the vagina and this could lead to urinary problems down the road. Surgery is the only thing that can repair this problem if it occurs. Many women do not experience these types of side effects, but doctors will see one occur here and there. In order to help the vagina become stronger without the cervix and uterus, doctors will suggest Kegel exercises. These can be done at any time and women can even do them while sitting at their desks at work!

There are a few health risks involved when a hysterectomy is suggested. Blood loss could happen during the surgery, as well as damage to the surrounding areas of the body. There is always the risk of infection and side effects or allergic reactions to the anesthesia. Every surgery may have complications of this nature and doctors will always go over these risks before the surgery begins.

Hysterectomies have long-term effects and short-term effects. They are a way to help women who have horrible pain during their periods. These women may also have heavy flows that keep them from their daily activities. When a hysterectomy is suggested by the doctor, it does mean that the woman's options have been weighed and the chances are that she is better off having the surgery than not at all. This procedure will eventually make her feel better and there will be no more painful and heavy periods for her to deal with.

Menopause and hysterectomies do not cure PCOS. They may change the symptoms up a little, but they will not make it go away. It is still important that women with PCOS take care of their bodies, exercise, and eat right no matter what. PCOS may also get worse as a woman enters menopause. The hormonal changes in her body can cause a lot of stress and emotions. It is important for women to remember that there are supplements and diets that can ease these side effects and symptoms.

Menopause changes a woman greatly and with PCOS, there can be more changes than usual. It is important to check in with a doctor about supplements during menopause and to see if they will help to combat PCOS as well. With the hormones and emotions running high, a doctor may be able to suggest ways to combat emotional and hormonal changes. There are plenty of natural supplements to help and some prescribed medications that can help a woman maintain her stress levels and her emotions as well.

Chapter 6: Birth Control and PCOS

Women with POCS have many options when it comes to using birth control. The hormones in birth control can actually help women balance their hormones if they have been diagnosed with PCOS. When a doctor prescribes birth control pills to women, it is important that they are aware of the side effects that they can have. Not every woman does want to be on birth control pills. Many women have said that the side effects made them feel terrible, so they chose other forms of contraception.

The side effects of birth control pills vary for every woman. Some women have noticed spotting during their periods. This will usually happen around the third month that a woman is on birth control. The pill is just as effective even though the woman is bleeding slightly. This seems to correct itself after a few months of taking the pill. If the bleed gets heavier or does not stop, it is clear that there is a problem and a doctor should be consulted.

Another side effect that birth control pills have is nausea. Some women who take the pill will begin to experience nausea when they first start taking it. These side effects will generally only last for a few weeks, but some women have noticed it for much longer. If the nausea does not go away within about three months, a doctor should be consulted. There could be other complications if this continues.

Breast tenderness can occur when the pill is being taken as well. There could also be some breast enlargement along with this tenderness. This will generally last a few weeks after beginning the pill. If the tenderness does continue for over a few weeks or lumps are found with it, it is very important to see a doctor as soon as possible. Breast tenderness could also be caused by having too much caffeine, too much salt, or wearing a bra that is too small or doesn't support the breasts properly.

Headaches and migraines are another reason that many women do not want to take birth control. It could cause both of these side effects and can make women miserable with the pain. The hormones in the pill can be the main cause of these headaches and they can trigger them rather quickly after taking the pill. Doctors can prescribe lower doses of birth control in order to make the risk of headaches lower. The headaches will get better, but if they continue to occur or they get worse, it is important to consult with a doctor.

Weight gain is another side effect that comes from taking birth control pills. This could be because of the fluid retention that may occur in the body when hormones are changing. This weight gain will happen around the breast and hip areas most of the time. Studies have been done on women who gained weight while taking birth control pills. The gained less than five pounds in about a six-month period. There are birth control pills that do contain fewer hormones that could help to keep the weight gain at bay.

One of the side effects that occur in most women on birth control is

a change in mood. Mood swings can be caused by the rising of hormones in the body and this can also increase the risk of depression and anxiety in women who are taking birth control pills. Once women begin to notice that their moods are changing, it is important that they consult with their medical doctor.

Along with mood swings, a lowering of the libido is also a side effect of birth control pills. This is another issue with changing the hormones in the body. When hormones are altered, a woman's sex drive can change dramatically and this can cause a lack of interest in sex or an increase in sexual desires. There are women who have noticed that their decreased libido was so bad that they had to find other methods of arousal to even be intimate with their partners. If birth control pills are causing this problem, it is time to talk with a doctor about them. There are some cases where birth control pills have caused the libido to increase so much that it also helped to reduce menstrual cramps, PMS, and uterine fibroids.

Vaginal discharge is another mild side effect that many women on birth control pills have encountered. There could be an increase in the vaginal fluids in the body, but some women have also seen a decrease in vaginal lubrication and this can cause very painful sex. Vaginal lubrication can be addressed by using lubricants during sex and that will help to have sex less painful and more comfortable. When the vaginal discharge occurs, it is not harmful at all. There may be some color changes in it and an odor could come from it as well. If a woman is very concerned about these changes, it is up to her to chat with her doctor about it.

Lastly, eye changes could be a side effect of taking birth control pills. Hormones have a lot to do with the body and as the body changes due to birth control pills, the eyes may change as well. Hormones can cause a thickening of the cornea. There haven't been many cases of this seen, but if it does occur, it simply means that wearing contact lenses may not be as comfortable as it once was. If women do wear contacts and have noticed this change, they should consult with their medical doctor and ophthalmologist about changes that they could make.

Birth control pills are not for every woman who needs contraception. The pill should not be taken by the following:

- pregnant women
- smokers who are 35 years old or over
- obese women
- women who take other medications
- women with heart problems or who have had a stroke
- women who have relatives that have had blood clots
- women with migraines
- women who have had breast cancer or diseases in the liver or gallbladder
- anyone who has had diabetes for over 20 years.

There are many warning signs that a woman's body should not be taking birth control pills. It is important that if these signs occur, a doctor is consulted immediately. The signs are as follows:

- stomach or abdominal pain
- chest pains or shortness of breath
- severe headaches and migraines
- blurred vision or loss of vision
- swelling or pains in the legs and thighs
- redness or swelling in the thighs or calves.

These factors could be a warning for a more serious condition.

Long-term Side Effects of Birth Control

There are plenty of reasons that women use birth control pills, but many women have long-term effects on them. These problems could start with cardiovascular issues. There could be an increase in heart attacks, strokes, and blood clots that come from changing of the hormones and taking birth control pills. All of these side effects are fatal so it is key to talk to a doctor if there has been any concern about these problems. Doctors can find the best solution for these problems if the patient has a family history of them.

When taking birth control pills, the risks of cancer can also increase. Because of the hormones in the female body, there could be some changes that occur while taking birth control. These changes could open the doors for more types of cancer to develop in the body, especially in the breasts or ovaries. There are types of birth control pills that use a lower hormone base than others. The cancers that are highest to spread in women who take birth control are breast cancer and ovarian cancer. These risks will become lower after about ten years of being off of the pill. These are the same risks that people have who have never taken the pill.

Women who have used birth control for longer amounts of time have been linked to having a very high risk of developing cervical cancer. HPV is one of the most common causes of cervical cancer, but it has not been linked to birth control pills. Liver cancer is another type of cancer that women who have taken birth control have a greater risk of getting. If women use birth control for over five years, their chances of getting liver cancer increase. It is important to consult with a medical doctor about any of these concerns before starting on birth control pills.

This talk of cancer and long-term side effects may sound terrifying, but there are many other forms of contraception that may not have any long-term side effects. It is always important to be aware of the alternatives and ways that will not change the hormone levels in the body.

Alternatives to Birth Control Pills

Birth control pills are not the right answer for every woman. In fact, many women just can't take the changing if their hormones, especially as they get older and experience more changes in their bodies, such as PCOS. The following are some birth control alternatives.

Condoms are a great place to start when it comes to unwanted pregnancy and STDs. Condoms are useful because they can stop sperm from coming into the egg during sex. This also helps men have some control over contraception as well. There are female condoms available on the market that has a ring at the end. This condom is placed into the woman's vagina. Condoms are pretty much available everywhere and they are generally made of latex. There are condoms made of other materials since some people do have an allergy to the latex. Lambskin is a great alternative to latex. There is only about an 18% risk that the condoms will not work.

Diaphragms are another contraceptive that women can use during intercourse. These are a dome-shaped cup that is inserted in the vagina to block the cervix. Diaphragms are used with spermicides to prevent sperm from meeting with the egg and causing pregnancy. There are a few disadvantages to using diaphragms though. They can cause urinary tract infections and irritation in the vagina. These irritations could be caused by the spermicide. Many women have found that they have a slight allergy to it. It is important that women know how to use a diaphragm correctly in order to keep from becoming pregnant. About six to thirteen pregnancies have occurred each year in about 100 women because they didn't know how to use the diaphragm properly.

The vaginal ring is another type of birth control that has become very popular lately. This is a plastic ring that is placed in the vagina. It releases hormones into the body to help suppress ovulation. Once a month, this ring is placed into the vagina for about three weeks. Then it is taken out for a week, while a woman has her menstrual period. This is very similar to taking birth control pills because the hormones are similar. Women can experience the same side effects from this ring as they do when they use the pill. Every year, there about ten pregnancies out of 100 women because the vaginal ring is used incorrectly. The side effects from the ring vary from headaches, lowered libido, and mood swings.

The intrauterine device, or IUD, is another contraceptive that is inserted into the body. These devices are made from copper and plastic. A doctor inserts the IUD into the uterus and they can contain hormones, although some do not. IUDs with hormones help to thicken the mucus in the cervix and keep ovulation from happening. Those without hormones help to make an inflammatory response to sperm inside of the uterus. This response is toxic to sperm and can keep a woman from becoming pregnant when it is inserted. The amazing benefit of IUDs is that they can last up to ten years once they have been inserted properly by a doctor. There have been very few cases of pregnancy in women with IUDs. There are some side effects from IUDs, just like other forms of birth control. Women have noted to have spotting and irregular periods, along with heavy periods and painful cramps.

Contraceptive implants can also be used as a form of birth control. These are small, plastic rods that are also implanted into the body. They are placed in the upper arm and this is a minor surgery that is done. These implants will release hormones for three years in a woman's body. They are used to help thicken the mucus around the cervix and helps to suppress ovulation. It has been shown that these implants are about 99.5% effective when it comes to birth control. There are some side effects as well. They include back pain, spotting, missed periods, and some higher risks of noncancerous ovarian cysts. These side effects did lessen after a few weeks of having the implant.

Sterilization is a permanent form of contraception. This surgery is generally done to the man in the partnership. It is used to block the tubes that transport sperm to the penis. When this surgery is done in woman, it is used to block the fallopian tubes. There are complications that can arise from sterilization. There could be infections, bruising, and lumps that develop in the tissue around the vas deferens in men.

Lastly, there are shots that can be given to women as a form of birth control. This is generally more reliable than the pill because it is done by the doctor and there is no pill to have to take daily. This is a hormonal type of birth control however. This type of birth control does bring side effects as well. The side effects are similar to those of birth control pills, such as headaches, spotting, and backaches. This shot does show increased chances of developing breast cancer, Chlamydia, and HIV. There are also some links to cardiovascular problems with the shot as well. Gaining weight may also be another side effect of this type of birth control. There are more advantages of the show because it does not need to be taken daily, it is given every three months. This shot is 99% effective as well.

Best Birth Control Pills for PCOS

PCOS is generally diagnosed in women who are still at the age of bearing children. Doctors do not have a cure for it as of yet, but there are ways to help combat the symptoms. One of these ways is by using birth control pills. The imbalance of hormones in women who have PCOS can be helped by taking birth control pills, but not all birth control pills will work for women with PCOS. Every symptom will vary from woman to woman but choosing the right birth control pill can help regulate the period and make it predictable for women who do want to conceive a child at some point.

How can birth control pills affect PCOS? Birth control pills can be hormonal or contain lower numbers of hormones. When birth control pills are hormonal, they will contain estrogen and progestin. When these hormones are combined, they help to regulate any imbalances that women may have. These pills can help in the case of hormone imbalances in women who do have PCOS. Most hormonal birth control pills are safe for all women, but there are women who have side effects from them. We have reviewed the side effects of birth control pills previously. Women with PCOS could encounter more side effects because of the changes it makes in a woman's body. There is a greater risk of diabetes in women with PCOS, the danger of blood clots in the legs, and greater chance of weight gain in women with PCOS. If women are obese, the chances of side effects from birth control pills do grow higher with PCOS.

There are quite a few birth control pills on the market today and doctors will be able to suggest the right one for women with PCOS. Combination birth control pills work well with women with PCOS. These pills work just like hormonal pills. There are a variety of these pills on the market today. The following is a list of combination birth control pills that work well with women who have PCOS:

- Alesse
- April
- Enpresse
- Estrostep
- Lessina
- Levora
- Loestrin
- Mircette

- Natazia
- Ortho-Novum
- Ortho Tri-Cyclen
- Yasmin
- Yaz

There are some birth control pills that have lower amounts of estrogen than others and many women choose these because of their hormonal imbalances. The lower estrogen pills can help to reduce the side effects of PCOS, but it is not a cure.

Women with very painful periods and PCOS have options for birth control pills that help them to find relief from their painful cramps. Many women choose to take birth control pills that give them fewer periods because of the pain of the periods. There are pills that can help with this such as:

- Lybrel
- Seasonique
- Seasonale

Minipills are also an option for women with PCOS. Women who often experience side effects from birth control pills are often given minipills. These pills are generally given to women who are smokers or obese.

Birth control pills do help to combat the symptoms of PCOS, but they are not a cure for it. There are many options for women to try when it comes to trying to fight off PCOS and it is important that they consult with their doctor before trying new diets or medications. Birth control pills can help women deal with PCOS and it is important that they know that birth control pills are not the only option when it comes to fighting the symptoms of PCOS.

Chapter 7: Research on PCOS

Why is PCOS such a complex disorder? Why is it so hard to find a cure and any research to get us closer to a cure? This disorder isn't new, it just hadn't been diagnosed in this way in the past. There needs to be more research done on women, but it has been extremely tough to get women to volunteer for these PCOS studies. Women don't find that they have much of a pay off when they volunteer for these types of studies. These studies would pay for all of the testing done on the women, but most of them don't want to spend a lot of time getting tested over and over again. Although, these tests could find the cure, many women just don't want to take any more tests than they have to. PCOS studies will also have women switch or stop taking their medications altogether. Many women don't want to give up their normal medication routines out of fear that the tests won't work on their PCOS symptoms.

In PCOS research, there has to be a lot of financial backing too. These studies are very expensive to hold and there is a lack of sponsors when it comes to researching PCOS. There are many other conditions that are the first to get financial backing because of the threat to society they have. PCOS has gotten less funding because the NIH feels there are other disorders that cause more economic burdens, morbidity, and impact on the quality of life.

PCOS is not a new disorder. In fact, it was first diagnosed by doctors in 1935. It was considered to be a very rare disorder at that time, but now about 10% of all women have it. While research is constantly being done on PCOS, it is still difficult to find a true cause of it. Knowledge of PCOS is not as widespread as many other disorders and that is why many women are finding it hard to get the help they need to combat the symptoms. Many women aren't even aware that they have PCOS. There are still areas of the world that do not have the doctors with knowledge of PCOS and they have no one to consult about their symptoms. Good resources are needed when it comes to fighting off a disorder like this, but if women are unaware of having it, it will not get any better for them and can ruin their chances of having a child.

We have discussed a lot of challenges doctors have when they go to diagnose PCOS. In women who are younger, around the age of puberty, it may be even more difficult to diagnose them because they are already having some changes in their hormones and bodies. Many of them are also having irregular periods and skin problems. These are all symptoms of PCOS, but they are also simple signs that a girl is entering puberty. This can be where it becomes incredibly difficult to diagnose PCOS properly. There are also challenges in diagnosing it in women who are going through menopause. Their hormone levels are also changing and this can be seen as a sign of PCOS and menopause. The challenges for diagnosing PCOS just seem to get higher and higher with no cure in sight for women with it.

Relationship Between AMH and PCOS

One way that doctors are trying to help women with PCOS is by focusing on what biomarkers can be helpful. One of these potential biomarkers is called Anti-Mullerian hormone or AMH. What is AMH? The Anti-Mullerian Hormone can be best described as a glycoprotein hormone that is related to activin and inhibin. It is a protein hormone that is very important in helping the development of the reproductive organs in a male fetus and it is helpful in keeping the ovaries and uterus healthy. It is produced by the testes and the ovaries in men and women.

AMH has quite the role in the reproductive organs and is present in both men and women. It can help to regulate sex steroid production during puberty and also in adults in the testes and ovaries. When it is present in the ovaries, it works wonders in the early stages of ovarian follicle development. When women are developing ovarian follicles, they will begin to support eggs during ovulation and fertilization. When a woman has more ovarian follicles, the more she will produce AMH in her ovaries. The AMH in her bloodstream can actually be measured by how many ovarian follicles are left in her ovaries. This is known as the ovarian reserve.

The ovarian reserve is a term used to describe the potential of a woman to reproduce and it is based on the number of eggs she has. It also takes into account the quality of her eggs. When women begin to age, the ovarian reserve begins to drop lower and lower. If a woman is diagnosed with PCOS, it could be a sign that she has a much lower ovarian reserve. This could be part of the reason for her infertility due to PCOS. Lower ovarian reserves can also be caused by smoking, genetics, radiation, and ovarian surgeries. PCOS can also have effects on the ovaries and the ovarian reserve. This has been something that many doctors and researchers have been looking into as well.

Is there such a thing as too much or too little AMH? Women can have too much AMH in their bodies and this can cause some side effects. The levels of AMH that a woman has can predict how women will respond if they are having in vitro fertilization. The levels of AMH in a woman get to their highest around puberty and will get lower when menopause begins. Higher levels of AMH have been associated with

PCOS, but tests are still being done on women to see just how much of an effect AMH has on PCOS diagnosis.

AMH has been given a lot of attention lately. It could be a substitute for ovarian imaging. It is being considered as a biomarker for women with PCOS because it has high concentrations of ovarian follicles. Because PCOS is characterized by hormone imbalances, AMH is part of the reason for these imbalances. There is clearly a relationship between PCOS and AMH.

As women begin to age, their hormones switch and change and are all over the place! Women with high levels of AMH will most likely be diagnosed with PCOS. How does a woman know her AMH levels? There are blood tests that are given to women who are curious about their AMH levels. These blood tests have been used as a very helpful way to help diagnose women with PCOS and help identify other hormone levels. Women who receive results of over 48 pmol/L, which stands for picomole per liter, have higher levels of AMH. This could be a sure sign of PCOS. About 98% of women who have a high count of AMH have been diagnosed positive for PCOS.

For women who are trying to get pregnant, there has been concern about how well fertility treatments work for those with higher levels of AMH. Are they able to receive these treatments and what are the chances that they will work? It is important that women know their hormone levels when they go into looking more at their fertility health. The healthier they are and the healthier their bodies are, the more successful fertility treatments will be. With high levels of AMH, there may be some questions that come up if the treatments will work and how quickly they will work. It seems that so far, women with PCOS have been reacting very positively to fertility treatments. In vitro fertilization has been the most successful for them, but there have been some cases where they worked too well and this caused ovarian hyperstimulation syndrome.

What is ovarian hyperstimulation syndrome? OHSS can affect women that have had hormone injections in order to help become pregnant. It will generally happen when women are using in vitro fertilization to get pregnant. OHSS can be caused when too much of the medication has gotten into the reproductive system. This causes the ovaries to be swollen and it is very painful. Some women with OHSS gain weight quickly, suffer from vomiting, and abdominal pain. OHSS can happen randomly to women who have never had fertilization treatments.

There are many symptoms of OHSS and they range from very mild to incredibly severe. The mild symptoms are abdominal pain, bloating, nausea, vomiting, and diarrhea. The severe symptoms include extreme weight gain of about 35 to 45 pounds in a week, severe pain in the abdomen, severe vomiting, blood clots in the legs, and enlarged abdomen. Any time a woman does experience these symptoms, it is important for her to see a doctor immediately. Having PCOS gives women a higher risk of developing OHSS.

Although PCOS and AMH are related, fertility treatments can help women who have higher levels of AMH. Once they are tested and their levels are determined, their doctors can work with them to find which fertility treatments work best.

PCOS and IVF

IVF, also known as in vitro fertilization, is one of the most successful ways for a woman to become pregnant. IVF is successful because it uses medications and different surgical procedures in order to help sperm to fertilize the woman's egg and then that egg is implanted into the uterus. Medication is taken at the beginning of the IVF process. This medication helps to mature the eggs and get them ready to be fertilized. The doctor will then take the eggs out of the woman's body. They will mix the eggs with sperm. This is done in a lab and the doctor will work on fertilizing the eggs with the sperm. When one egg has been fertilized, they will place the egg into the uterus. Pregnancy will then happen if the embryos implant into the uterus.

When women begin IVF, there are many steps that they have to follow. Sometimes this can take months at a time to accomplish. Some women get lucky and they get pregnant on the first try. This is not typical though. Generally it takes more than one try to become pregnant with IVF. If women are having fertility problems, IVF can help to increase the chances of a woman becoming pregnant. IVF is not guaranteed for all women. There are many women who were not able to become pregnant with IVF and had to seek other means of fertility treatment.

The IVF process can be very complex, but when a woman's doctor takes the time to explain it to her properly, it becomes easier to understand. When it begins, as we mentioned, the woman begins to take medications to get her eggs ready to be fertilized. This is the process called ovulation induction. There are regular blood tests and ultrasounds done during this time. These tests will measure the hormone levels and make sure that eggs are being produced. These eggs will then be used for fertilization.

When eggs have been produced and the doctor thinks that there enough to try to fertilize, they will extract the eggs from the body. This is called egg retrieval and is a minor surgery. Egg retrieval is done by putting a tube through the vagina and into the ovaries. This is where the eggs are held. There is a needle that is connected to the tube and it works like a vacuum to extract the eggs. This is done gently, but medication is given to help patients remain calm and in little pain.

After the eggs have been extracted, the doctor will begin the sperm and egg combining process in the lab. This is called insemination. The eggs and sperm are kept together and fertilization will happen while they are being mixed. The sperm is injected into the eggs because once they are out, they have little motility. This is why the doctor has to help them to find the egg. Soon, the eggs will become embryos.

It takes about three to five days after the egg retrieval for the embryos to start to form. Then they can be placed into the uterus of the patient. This process is called embryo transfer. The embryo is inserted with the help of a small tube that goes into the cervix and uterus. This is another minor surgery and is not very painful. How does a woman get pregnant in this way? When the embryos attach to the uterus, pregnancy occurs.

It is important to know that when the embryo transfer happens, a woman needs to take a full day to rest her body. The embryo needs time to find its way to the uterus so resting the body is the best way to make sure it happens. Some doctors will suggest a woman taking hormone pills for the first few weeks after the embryo transfer has been done. These hormones will make it much easier for the embryo to make it and form a baby.

IVF does have some side effects however. Women can have signs such as bloating, tender breasts, mood swings, migraines, bruising, allergic reactions to medication, and bleeding. If the side effects are too much to handle, it is important that a woman talks with her doctor about them. A side effect that is not medical is the emotional difficulty involved in IVF. These procedures can be taxing on a person's physical and emotional status. Many IVF families will have depression and anxiety during the whole process. Getting pregnant isn't easy for everyone, so it does take its toll on patients and their partners.

Many women decide to try methods other than IVF because it is pretty expensive. Many states have laws that women who want to use IVF must have health insurance that will cover fertility drugs. There are quite a few insurance companies that will not cover any of these fees. This is why it gets expensive. Many insurance companies feel that this is not a necessary medical expense so they choose not to cover it. The fees are incredibly high and the first cycle of IVF can end up costing over $15,000! That includes blood tests, ultrasounds, lab work, and the storing of embryos. This is not exactly something a lot of people can afford easily.

When women have been diagnosed with PCOS, it is important that they weigh their options when it comes to getting pregnant. Because PCOS has a very negative effect on how women get pregnant, they may look into fertility treatments such as IVF. For women who have PCOS, IVF has about a 60% chance of working. Seeing an IVF specialist is the best way to go about finding more information about becoming pregnant with PCOS.

Other Fertility Treatments for Women with PCOS

IVF is one of the most popular fertility treatments for women who are trying to get pregnant. Women with PCOS have much lower chances of getting pregnant naturally so it is important that they find a treatment that will work best for them. IVF is pretty expensive, but there are many other types of treatments that can work for women who are trying to conceive a child.

When looking for the perfect fertility treatment to get pregnant, women must first go through a variety of tests that will help doctors to find out what treatment is the best choice for them. These tests will check different hormone levels and the health of their eggs. There are tests to check ovulation cycles, condition of the fallopian tubes, ovarian reserves, and imaging tests that will take a look at the pelvic area for signs of ovarian diseases. Doctors will also ask questions about the health of the patient. They will focus on what is causing infertility, how long they have been infertile, and how old they are. They will ask questions about their partner as well in order to find the best way to treat infertility.

There are some types of infertility that cannot be repaired so doctors will ask quite a few questions and conduct many tests. This may seem intrusive at first, but if a woman truly wants to get pregnant, she must be aware of these tests. Women can be treated for infertility through IVF, fertility drugs, intrauterine insemination, and surgery to restore fertility.

Fertility drugs are usually the first method of getting pregnant for women with PCOS. The way that these drugs work is that they are given to women who want to get pregnant and these drugs will stimulate ovulation or help to regulate ovulation. These drugs are used for women with ovulation disorders or other disorders such as PCOS. These drugs work because they act as natural hormones in a woman's body. They will stimulate the hormones that help to trigger ovulation. If the drugs work, ovulation is stimulated and the woman has a much higher chance of getting pregnant. The drugs can also help women to produce more eggs at one time.

There are many types of fertility drugs. Clomiphene citrate is one that women can take orally. This pill helps to stimulate ovulation and makes the pituitary gland make more FSH and LH. These hormones can stimulate growth in the ovaries and produce eggs. This medication is in the category called ovulatory stimulants. It works much like estrogen in the woman's body does. This is why it is often suggested for women who are trying to become pregnant. The brand names of this pill are Clomid, Milophene, and Serophene.

Gonadotropins are a type of fertility drug that doctors suggest for women who are struggling to get pregnant. The name of this drug comes from the stimulation of the gonads in women and men. In women, they are called ovaries. This is a thyroid-stimulating hormone that helps women to produce more LH and FSH. This can help to regulate the functions of the ovaries. FHS, also known as follicle-stimulating hormone, helps to mature the eggs in a woman's body. This can help to stimulate ovulation and that helps a woman to become pregnant. These hormones have various names such as Menopur, Ovidrel, Pregnyl, HCG, Novarel, Chorex, and Fertinex. These hormones can only be prescribed by a doctor.

Metformin is a drug that is commonly prescribed to women with PCOS who are trying to get pregnant. It is used to help the blood sugar levels in the body. Because women with PCOS are at a higher risk of developing diabetes, this medication is used to help them with insulin levels. Insulin levels and diabetes can also cause problems with fertility so this is one of the reasons that doctors prescribe this drug to women with PCOS.

Letrozole is another drug that has been known to help women with PCOS become pregnant. Letrozole is known for inducing ovulation. It has also been used for chemotherapy and women who have breast cancer. It can help to slow down breast cancer and does change the amount of estrogen in the body. It helps women get pregnant by making ovulation occur quicker and more often than usual.

Lastly, there is Bromocriptine. This is a drug that is helpful to women and their sexual functions. It is known for treating infertility, regulation of menstrual periods, and low hormone levels. This is prescribed commonly to women who have PCOS and are trying to get pregnant. With diet and exercise, this drug works really well for women who want to become pregnant. Just like other pills, it has side effects that do need to be discussed with a doctor if they occur on a regular basis.

These medications are all available to women who are looking for a way to become pregnant. Many women with PCOS are candidates for medications, but some women will seek other methods of fertilization treatments. Some of these treatments are surgical.

Fertilization Surgeries for Women with PCOS

Fertility surgery is an option for women with PCOS who have found that they cannot get pregnant by any other means. When a woman's doctor tells her that her options for medication are limited, surgery is the next best option. There are quite a few types of fertility surgeries for women today. They can all be done in a hospital and generally they are quick and do not require the woman to stay overnight at the hospital. There are specific situations and symptoms that doctors will suggest having surgery. These vary from woman to woman, but there are generally uterine fibroids, pelvic adhesions, polyps, and endometriosis.

The first of these fertility surgeries is called laparoscopy. This is a surgery that is done by the woman's doctor and it is said to be one of the most successful surgeries for fertility problems. This surgery is not too invasive to women and it can be done as an outpatient surgery. Laparoscopy uses very small cuts in order to put a small camera into the body. The camera is called a laparoscope and it can look into the body to see just where the fertility problems are. This surgery has been used for many other types of conditions such as gallbladder surgery.

This surgery uses small cuts that are about half an inch long. It is often called keyhole surgery. When it is used for fertility problems, this surgery is called female pelvic laparoscopy. The doctor will get a chance to view the reproductive organs in their patient. This surgery can find any causes of infertility problems in a woman's body, it can examine larger tissue masses such as cysts or polyps, confirms endometriosis, and can check for any problems that are in the fallopian tubes. If the doctors have found a blockage in the fallopian tubes and this could be one of the main causes for infertility.

When getting ready for this surgery, it is important to know what to expect. During the surgery, the patient will be given a general anesthetic to keep them from feeling any pain. The incision for the camera is made near the navel. There is generally a second incision made near the pubic hairline. The doctor will use the camera for a few minutes to see what they can find inside the woman's reproductive organs. Once everything has been viewed and the doctor has a clear idea of what needs to be done, the patient will be in recovery for about an hour. They will then be able to fully recover at home for some rest and relaxation. In practically every surgery like this one, patients are only at the hospital for about three to four hours. There are rare cases that a patient will have to stay overnight with this surgery. Women who have had this surgery are asked to check in with their doctors in order to make sure that they have healed properly.

This surgery can help doctors to determine the fertility problems in women, but there are some risks in having it as well. This is a very safe surgery overall, but there have been cases where women have had side effects or problems. Only about three out of 1,000 women have had any complications though. Some women experienced injuries to the organs nearby and have had bleeding or bloating. Women who have allergy reactions to anesthesia often have complications as well.

Hysteroscopic surgery is another type of female fertility surgery known to help women with PCOS and other infertility issues. This type of surgery is used to help check the size and lining of the uterus. This surgery can also check for abnormalities that can cause infertility and miscarriages. This surgery works by implanting a small tool into the vagina. It will go through the cervix and the uterus. There is a camera on this tool that can give the doctor a better view of the uterus. This is used to diagnose any problems that the woman may have with her uterus or fertility.

The doctor may use these results to find out if there are polyps or tumors in the uterus. They can find out just what is causing the woman to have fertility problems and the health of the fallopian tubes. These surgeries can actually be done in the doctor's office. This is one of the best ways to help to diagnose any fertility problems in a woman.

There are a few risks with this surgery as well. The most common problem is bleeding, blood clotting problems, and severe allergic reactions. There have also been serious complications in the lungs of patients. These complications are not life-threatening and can be contained by the doctor doing the surgery.

Tubal surgery is another type of fertility surgery for women. If a woman has tried everything to get pregnant, there could be a blockage in the fallopian tubes. This means that she will need to have surgery to correct this blockage. Tubal surgery is just the right thing to correct it. There could also be infections in the body that have caused these blockages. Ectopic pregnancy is another problem that women may have and need to have surgery to repair this problem.

The fallopian tubes in a woman connect to the ovaries and the uterus. When women are trying to conceive, sperm will swim to the vagina through the cervix and uterus. The fallopian tubes will then lead the sperm to the egg where it can be fertilized and the woman can become pregnant. If the fallopian tubes are blocked, they will not be able to become pregnant and tubal surgery is needed to repair the blockage.

There are many reasons that the fallopian tubes could be blocked or have problems. What many people do not know is that STDs can cause fertility problems to show up years after they have been diagnosed and they could be the culprit for any fallopian tube blockages or problems. Chlamydia and gonorrhea are two of the most common STDs that can cause blockages in the fallopian tubes. Tuberculosis is also known to cause these blockages and can also cause damages to the fallopian tubes.

After having a tubal surgery, the chances of pregnancy do rise quite a bit. When women have tubal surgeries, their doctors will do a lot of monitoring of their fallopian tubes. There are a few risks for complications, but as long as they are being monitored, chances are they can become pregnant much quicker. There may be some cases of vaginal bleeding and abdominal pain, but these are completely normal after having this surgery.

IUI or intrauterine insemination is another type of fertility surgery. This is a treatment that involves using surgery to implant sperm into the female's uterus. There is one goal of IUI and it is to make a woman become pregnant. This is a way to give the sperm a head start to the egg in order to make a woman pregnant. This is a less invasive surgery and is less expensive than having in vitro fertilization surgery.

IUI is often used for unexplained infertility, repairing cervix lining problems, helping to repair cervical scar tissue, and dysfunction when trying to become pregnant. There are women who should not have this surgery, such as women with fallopian tube blockages or infections, women with pelvic infections, and women who have severe endometriosis. IUI works in many ways to help women to become pregnant. Before this surgery, women are given fertility medications and are monitored by their doctor. These medications help to stimulate the ovulation cycle and are used until the eggs become mature inside of the woman. The IUI surgery will then take place about 36 hours after they have started to take the medication.

This process only takes about 20 minutes to perform and doesn't give the woman that much discomfort when it happens. Once it is completed, the doctor and the woman will simply wait and watch for signs that they have become pregnant.

IUI is very successful when it comes to helping to get women to conceive a child. There is about a 20% success rate per woman per cycle. This is quite high especially for women who have had problems conceiving for years. Because this surgery is less invasive and expensive than IVF, many women will choose to have it. The pregnancy rates are also lower than in IVF so women may have to attempt pregnancy with this surgery more than once. This could become pricey in the long run.

Another type of fertility treatment is called embryo cryopreservation. This is the process of freezing and storing a woman's embryos. This is one part of the in vitro process. The embryos are stored for as long as the woman wants them to stay. Once the woman is ready to become pregnant, she can have them thawed out and they can be used to help her become pregnant. This is a very popular treatment and there are currently hundreds of thousands of embryos stored today.

Women may choose this treatment because they have had embryos destroyed and need a new way to conceive a child. This treatment can help give women a chance to have a baby after trying every other method. If IVF does fail for women the first time, this is a way to try again with the same embryos as before. If a couple does end up having a baby through this process, they can actually use their embryos to help them to have another baby. These embryos can actually be used and donated to other women who are trying to have children. These embryos can also be donated for research purposes. In fact, many women with PCOS have started to donate their embryos in order to help researchers find a cure for the disorder.

How does this process work? The embryos are frozen and stored in a slow freezing method. The embryos are frozen in different stages. This helps to protect the embryos and when they are slowly cooled, it helps them from losing the possibility of becoming a baby at some point. When they are frozen completely, they are kept at about -321 degrees Fahrenheit. This process is called vitrification and will help to keep the cells and embryos safe for fertilization. When the woman is ready to use them, they can be slowly thawed out and then placed in special fluids where the cells are completely restored. Once the embryos have been thawed, they can be used to fertilize and hopefully they will become a child for the woman.

Fertility surgeries, treatments, and drugs can all help women with PCOS to become pregnant. These treatments are helpful for women who know that they want to have a child. Once they have started these treatments, they have a much higher chance of becoming pregnant.

Conclusion

PCOS is a disorder that many women have been diagnosed with and now have no idea how it can be cured. This is a lifetime disorder, but why is it affecting more and more women each year? There have been many studies done so far about PCOS and how it affects every woman who is diagnosed with it. These women all have different experiences when it comes to their health and their diagnosis. These symptoms can actually have long-term effects on their physical and mental health.

Mood swings and disorders can occur when women have developed PCOS. This can cause a decrease in the quality of life for women with PCOS. The mood swings can cause anxiety and depression and a decrease in sexual satisfaction and libido. These changes in women can cause horrible emotional problems in them. Many women who have PCOS have had thoughts of suicide and it is now being called the silent disorder that can kill.

PCOS puts a woman's body through so many changes. It is no wonder that it makes women feel emotionally wrecked and tired. The emotional toll that it takes on women has not been talked about much in this book and we wanted to educate our readers on just what it can do to women. When women are trying to have a baby, their emotions are all over the place. When they go into their doctor's office, only to hear they have PCOS and possibly infertility, it takes another toll on them. They are curious about why it is happening to them and just what they can do about it. There is not much they can do actually and when they hear this, the emotions can go through the roof. Many doctors say that they see an "emotional fall out" when the words are uttered. Women with PCOS suffer from weight gain, hormone imbalances, and infertility. All of these symptoms make it incredibly difficult for women with PCOS to even get up in the morning. Why is it going so unnoticed though?

Most women with PCOS have started struggling with body image problems and the symptoms don't help their cause. When they begin to grow hair on their face and lose hair on their heads, they begin to think of themselves in a different way. This way is not as positive as they would like it to be, but with all of these hormonal changes, who knows what they are really going through? A lot of body shaming comes from this stage in a woman's PCOS life as well. When the average person looks at a woman with PCOS, they don't know her situation. They don't know the reason for the extra hair on her face and this could turn into body shaming. Once the body-shaming begins, the depression hits and when the depression hits, a woman could have thoughts of suicide. PCOS does have quite a few links to mental health and we want to show our readers exactly what can happen when a woman has been diagnosed with PCOS.

Women with PCOS are at a much greater risk of becoming depressed or dealing with other mental health problems. Another problem that women with PCOS face are having an eating disorder. Why would they develop this? Think about the weight gain that happens when PCOS occurs. Women with it need to lose weight in order to conceive a child, so their chances of developing an eating disorder are very high.

These mental health problems can also be caused by changes in their hormones. When women are exposed to higher levels of male hormones, which happens regularly with PCOS, they have a higher risk of developing mental health issues. When women are diagnosed with PCOS, they have a higher chance of developing depression that they can't just shake off. This is more than just being sad about having PCOS, this is serious depression. The types of depression that women with PCOS develop need to be treated medically and by a therapist.

Women with PCOS can develop a major depressive disorder. This is a form of depression that lasts for many weeks and sometimes months. This type of depression takes women away from the activities that they love to do daily. They will sleep all day and most of the time, they will blow off any important tasks that they have to do. They will make it to work, but their job may suffer in the meantime. They will have lowered energy levels and they will lose any interest in pleasure or sex. This is seen very often in women who have been diagnosed with PCOS. It becomes difficult for women with PCOS to motivate themselves. Women with this type of depression will need to find the right therapist to chat with them about how to get through this depression.

Bipolar depression is another type of mental illness that women with PCOS are often diagnosed with. There are a few types of bipolar disorder. The first is bipolar I and it is often called manic depression. This is when a woman has experienced manic episodes and their mood is elevated and they act in an erratic fashion. Bipolar II disorder is different because it has symptoms that impair the woman who is diagnosed. These symptoms will last up to a week and there is irritability added to the mood swings. These symptoms are not as severe as bipolar I.

Seasonal affective disorder is another type of depression that women may be diagnosed with if they also have PCOS. This type of depression will generally take place at the same time each year. Most women will fall into this depression when it gets cold and gray outside. The days are much shorter at this time and women exhibit a lack of energy and get tired easily. Generally, seasonal affective disorder gets better when the sun shines longer and the days get brighter.

How do women know that they have signs of depression? There are quite a few and with women with PCOS, they could show up much stronger than with other women. Here are a few symptoms of depression in women with PCOS:

- Fatigue
- Feeling sadness constantly
- Feeling lonely
- Feeling helpless
- Crying uncontrollably
- Insomnia
- No motivation or energy
- Changes in weight
- Guilty feelings
- Trouble concentrating

- No interest in sex
- No interest in hobbies
- Terrible decision making
- Migraines
- Digestive problems

Depression can be treated in many ways and when women with PCOS have been diagnosed with it, it is important that they find the help that they need. The first way to treat depression is by seeing a therapist. Therapists can help women with depression because they can hear them out. They can find out more about what is causing this depression and these feelings of dread and self-doubt. They can talk about the PCOS diagnosis and just how hard they are trying to have a child. Therapists are pretty easy to find and can help women retrain their brains to thinking more positive about life and PCOS. There is talk therapy, cognitive behavioral therapy, and interpersonal therapy.

Support groups are another great place for women to reach out to others. By searching for groups in their community, women with PCOS and depression may be able to find the right places to go. PCOS groups are popping up all over as well so these women may have more than one place to go when they are feeling self-doubt and shame. These PCOS support groups can help women to get through the feelings that they are having. These groups teach women how to cope and can even help them to change their lives.

Medication seems to be the most popular way to find treatment for depression. Antidepressants are the most popular. There are several types of antidepressants that can treat women. Some of these antidepressants may have side effects that could affect a woman's reproductive health, so it is important that women find the right medication for their depression.

Self-Esteem Problems with PCOS

Depression is just one of the horrible side effects of having PCOS. Self-esteem problems are another. For the women that suffer from PCOS, it can be very taxing on their self-esteem. The weight gain, unwanted hair, and infertility all have quite the effect on women that have PCOS.

Each woman that has been diagnosed with PCOS will have different symptoms, but there is one thing that all of these women have in common and that is loss of self-esteem and confidence in themselves. Many women have issues with infertility with PCOS and the ones who are trying to have a family may experience much lower rates in self-esteem than those who are not trying to have a baby. A woman's self-esteem has a lot to do with how she feels about herself and if she cannot give her partner a baby, this could crush her and cause her to not love herself the way that she used to.

PCOS can cause a lot of masculine traits to occur to women. A lot of women cannot take the extra hair growing on their faces and losing the hair on their head. This can make them feel less like a woman and can be a huge factor when it comes to destroying their self-esteem. If women are single and have PCOS, this may cause them to not want to get out and date. They may be afraid that the hairs on their chin will show up on their date and this could ruin their entire evening. Doctors have heard it all and there are ways to help, but this is one of the results of PCOS. There are medications that can be taken for excess hair on the body and for hair loss. If acne breakouts occur along with extra hair, there are medications for that as well.

The weight factor is a major self-esteem destroyer. Obesity is something that many people look down upon and critique. This is why it can be very difficult for women with PCOS to handle weight gain. Women often feel judged by the way they look and how much they weigh. This takes quite a toll on the self-esteem of women who have PCOS. Many women also feel that they are discriminated against because of their weight so this can stop them from accomplishing even more in their lives than women who are at an average weight. This causes so many self-esteem and emotional problems that doctors may not even see in their patients until it's too late.

Infertility can really cause difficulties in the self-esteem of a woman. Many women think that if they cannot get pregnant and give their partner a child, they aren't enough woman for them. This is a soul-crushing reminder of how women are the ones who are supposed to carry the child and give birth to it. These are constant reminders to many women that they are not as feminine as they should be. This can not only cause self-esteem problems, but it can cause problems in a marriage as well. If the couple feels that they cannot conceive together, it could start many marriage problems that could lead to a divorce.

What can doctors do about these feelings of low self-esteem in their PCOS patients? First, women with PCOS need to realize that this is a condition that needs to be treated and not ignored. Many women are diagnosed with it and simply choose to ignore the medications, diet, exercise, and overall lifestyle change. Many women will not admit that they do have it and this can make it even worse for them.

Therapy does wonders for women who have low self-esteem due to PCOS. When women begin to have low self-esteem, they may be fighting depression and anxiety. We have talked about the ways to treat depression and we hope that women with PCOS will take their condition seriously so they can find the help that they need.

PCOS And Relationships

We have covered quite a bit in this book and we want our readers to know that there is one final issue to discuss when it comes to PCOS. It not only affects the woman, but it can affect her relationship and partner as well. PCOS should be discussed with her partner and the changes that her body is going through because of PCOS.

PCOS is frustrating and it can be an emotional ride for the woman. It can also affect relationships with spouse, friends, and family. It all starts with self-esteem issues and the changes that the body is going through. Irregular periods and difficulties in getting pregnant can cause stress in the home. These changes can also lower self-esteem of a woman and that can cause her not to feel as sexy and loved as she once did. This can cause changes in her sex life and her partner could suffer from this as well. If a woman doesn't feel comfortable in her own skin, chances are, she will not want to even try to have a baby anymore. This is the sad truth about how PCOS can affect her self-esteem.

Relationships with friends and family could begin to suffer as well. Women may not want to see their friends anymore because of how they look. Friends will always be around to pick a woman up if she is going through these problems. It is up to the woman to be open about her condition and the changes that are happening in her body. Any good friend will realize that they need to step it up and help her out no matter what.

If the weight gain is the biggest issue, a woman can see a registered dietician for some help losing weight. They can write out a new diet plan for the woman and teach them some exercises that will help them lose the weight they need to. Women with PCOS who have gained a lot of weight may be that they can't hang out with their skinnier friends anymore. They may feel like they have failed because they have gained so much weight. Women with PCOS can change their diet and lifestyle to begin to lose weight and get their self-esteem higher. In fact, they may be able to call their friends and ask them to go to the gym with them or go hiking with them. There are so many ways for women with PCOS to lose weight that all they have to do is try.

Intimacy may begin to suffer as women with PCOS gain weight, develop acne, and grow excessive hair on the body. Women may not want their partner to see these changes and may not want to get naked in front of them anymore. This can be a terrible problem especially when it comes to the two of them wanting to have a family. Many women with PCOS have taken their relationship to a therapist where the two of them can talk to someone who can understand what they are both going through. This therapist can help both of them to better understand what PCOS is doing to the woman and her self-esteem.

When consulting with a sex or relationship therapist, it can put the couple in a rough spot. Not everyone wants a complete stranger to know what their sex life is like. This could possibly take a huge toll on the relationship. The therapist may also have to direct the couple to the right times to have sex in order to conceive. This is another issue that many couples have. They don't want someone to dictate when and where they have sex in order to have a baby. This will present challenges too. It is important that the woman with PCOS is open with her partner about what is happening in her body. When she is ready to contact a therapist, the couple must shop around for one together and see which one is best for the both of them.

Infertility may make things really hard for the relationship, but it doesn't have to ruin the partnership. This may cause some intimacy problems at the beginning, but it doesn't have to be what ruins the relationship. All relationships do take work, but when PCOS and infertility are involved, there may be a lot more work to do. If a couple wants to continue in their relationship, they will do whatever it takes in order to make the relationship truly work. They need to make sure that they make time for each other every day. With busy lives and work schedules, it can be incredibly tough to make this time together. This could be terrible for their relationship. This is why having dates each week could be helpful to reconnect the couple and get their love growing again.

If PCOS is really affecting a relationship, the couple needs to do whatever they can in order to help save it. If they want to have a child, they will need to be on the same page and know what the other is thinking about the situation. Having a child is a big step and having PCOS can just add to the stress of it all. This is why couples need to stick together through this tough time.

Getting diagnosed with PCOS isn't the end of the world. Many women may see it as that way, but there are many ways to help fight the symptoms and live a normal life again. Doctors have so many ways that they can now help women with PCOS and now, research is getting closer and closer to finding a cure and even a way to keep PCOS from spreading.

Only time will tell how much science can do for PCOS, but we are very positive about the outcomes. We know that it may be many years before we see a cure, but if they do single out the genes that cause PCOS, things will be looking up in no time at all! Women with PCOS will have to continue their current treatments until science finds a cure for them.

PCOS doesn't have to stop life. It can actually give women a new lease on life to get their weight and diet under control. It can help them to make some healthier choices for food and even some better choices for themselves. Getting diagnosed with PCOS doesn't end life, in fact, it could be just the beginning of a wonderful one!

www.ingramcontent.com/pod-product-compliance
Lightning Source LLC
Chambersburg PA
CBHW031155020426
42333CB00013B/683